AF750992

Surgical Techniques and Procedures

Edited by Georgios Tsoulfas

Published in London, United Kingdom

Surgical Techniques and Procedures
http://dx.doi.org/10.5772/intechopen.1006227
Edited by Georgios Tsoulfas

Contributors
Alessandro Maraschi, Andreea Pruteanu, Athina-Zacharoula Ditsiou, Gergo Jozsa, Ioana Păvăleanu, Konstantinos Ditsios, Kunal Bhakhri, Marcell Varga, Mustafa Karaağaç, Razvan Socolov, Thomas Fraccalini, Toma Bogdan, Toma Loredana, Triantafyllos Katsimentzas, Tripti Sinha, Tudor Butureanu, Vasileios Balamotis, Visar Disha

© The Editor(s) and the Author(s) 2025

The rights of the editor(s) and the author(s) have been asserted in accordance with the Copyright, Designs and Patents Act 1988. All rights to the book as a whole are reserved by INTECHOPEN LIMITED. The book as a whole (compilation) cannot be reproduced, distributed or used for commercial or non-commercial purposes without INTECHOPEN LIMITED's written permission. Enquiries concerning the use of the book should be directed to INTECHOPEN LIMITED rights and permissions department (permissions@intechopen.com).

Violations are liable to prosecution under the governing Copyright Law.

Individual chapters of this publication are distributed under the terms of the Creative Commons Attribution 4.0 License which permits commercial use, distribution and reproduction of the individual chapters, provided the original author(s) and source publication are appropriately acknowledged. If so indicated, certain images may not be included under the Creative Commons license. In such cases users will need to obtain permission from the license holder to reproduce the material. More details and guidelines concerning content reuse and adaptation can be found at http://www.intechopen.com/copyright-policy.html.

Notice

Statements and opinions expressed in the chapters are these of the individual contributors and not necessarily those of the editors or publisher. No responsibility is accepted for the accuracy of information contained in the published chapters. The publisher assumes no responsibility for any damage or injury to persons or property arising out of the use of any materials, instructions, methods or ideas contained in the book.

First published in London, United Kingdom, 2025 by IntechOpen
IntechOpen is the global imprint of INTECHOPEN LIMITED, registered in England and Wales, registration number: 11086078, 167-169 Great Portland Street, London, W1W 5PF, United Kingdom

For EU product safety concerns: IN TECH d.o.o., Prolaz Marije Krucifikse Kozulić 3, 51000 Rijeka, Croatia, info@intechopen.com or visit our website at intechopen.com.

British Library Cataloguing-in-Publication Data
A catalogue record for this book is available from the British Library

Surgical Techniques and Procedures
Edited by Georgios Tsoulfas
p. cm.
Print ISBN 978-1-83634-593-0
Online ISBN 978-1-83634-592-3
eBook (PDF) ISBN 978-1-83634-594-7

If disposing of this product, please recycle the paper responsibly.

IntechOpen
intechopen.com

Built by scientists, for scientists

Explore all IntechOpen books

Meet the editor

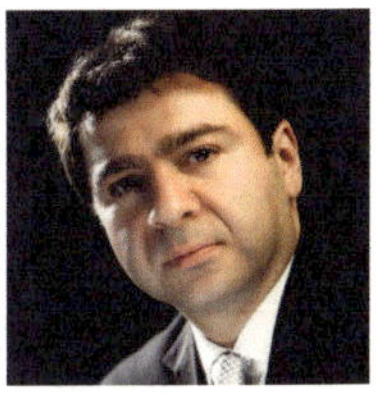

Dr. Georgios Tsoulfas received his MD from Brown University School of Medicine and completed a general surgery residency at the University of Iowa Hospitals and Clinics, as well as a transplant research fellowship at the Starzl Transplant Institute at the University of Pittsburgh. He then completed a two-year fellowship in transplantation surgery at Massachusetts General Hospital, an institution affiliated with Harvard Medical School, and subsequently joined the Division of Solid Organ Transplantation and Hepatobiliary Surgery at the University of Rochester Medical Center as an Assistant Professor of Surgery. He moved back to Greece in 2008, where he is currently a Professor of Transplantation Surgery and the Chief of the Department of Transplantation Surgery at the Aristotle University of Thessaloniki School of Medicine and the Center for Research and Innovation in Solid Organ Transplantation. He has published over 200 papers in peer-reviewed journals and PubMed, as well as 35 book chapters, with an H-index of 34 and an i10-index of 82, and has received over 7,500 citations. He has edited 8 books and serves as a reviewer for 30 international journals, as well as on the Editorial Board of several others, including International Surgery and Annals of Surgical Oncology. The recipient of awards such as the Edward E. Mason Award for excellence in patient care and education, he is a member of several professional organizations, including the TTS, Society of Surgical Oncology, the American Society of Transplant Surgeons, Association for Academic Surgery, International College of Surgeons, American College of Surgeons, International Liver Transplantation Society, Society for Laparoscopic Surgeons and International Hepato-Pancreato Biliary Association. He is also the recipient of the American College of Surgeons International Guest Scholarship. He has served as a member of multiple committees, including the International Relations Committee of the American College of Surgeons and the International Relations Committee of the American HepaticoPancreaticoBiliary Association (AHPBA). Currently the president of the Greek Chapter of the International College of Surgeons, he has also served as World President of the International College of Surgeons and as Chair of the International Relations Committee of the American College of Surgeons. He has served as a member of the AHPBA and the IHPBA Education and Training Committees, the E-AHPBA Education Committee (Training Program Accreditation), the ASTS CME and Professional Development Committee and the AASLD Training and Workforce Committee. He is also a member of the Executive Council of the Hellenic Surgical Society and President of the Hellenic Transplantation Society. Clinical and research interests include hepatobiliary surgery, primary and secondary hepatic malignancies, ischemia/reperfusion injury, and solid organ transplantation, as well as medical and surgical education and the application of technology, including artificial intelligence and 3D printing in surgery.

Contents

Preface

The complex nature of the surgery, which involves pre- and post-operative preparation and follow-up of the patient, in addition to the technical aspects, is an excellent example of the need for various specialities to collaborate in order to achieve the best possible outcome for the patient. In this book, the authors offer descriptions not only of the surgical and technical challenges and difficulties but also of the importance of preparing properly for various complications, as well as how to address them should they occur.

This book provides an overview of all the above, with chapters presenting challenges in various surgical specialities and offering us the distilled experience of the authors.

Overall, this book should be a valuable resource for any physician, whether in training or practice, who treats patients with surgical diseases.

Georgios Tsoulfas
Professor of Transplantation Surgery,
Chief of the Department of Transplantation Surgery,
Center for Research and Innovation in Solid Organ Transplantation,
Aristotle University School of Medicine,
Thessaloniki, Greece

Section 1

Minimally Invasive Surgery

Chapter 1

Robotic Innovations in Thoracic Surgery: State of the Art and Future Perspectives

Alessandro Maraschi, Thomas Fraccalini and Kunal Bhakhri

Abstract

This chapter examines the profound impact of robotic technology on thoracic surgery, emphasizing current innovations and future prospects. We begin with a brief historical overview of robotic systems, focusing on their evolution from the early models to Intuitive da Vinci platforms and the latest advancements in surgical robotics. The core of our analysis is the comparative effectiveness of robotic-assisted thoracic surgery (RATS) against traditional video-assisted thoracic surgery (VATS) and open surgery techniques. Key benefits of RATS discussed include enhanced surgical precision, minimized patient trauma, and improved clinical outcomes, such as decreased hospitalization times and enhanced lymph node harvesting. Further, the chapter delves into the integration of robotics in surgical training, highlighting the role of features such as dual-console setups. We explore ongoing technological advancements, such as the incorporation of artificial intelligence and improved imaging techniques, which are set to expand the capabilities and efficiency of RATS. We assess the potential of emerging robotic platforms and the implications of their features, such as single-port access and AI-driven tools, for the future of thoracic procedures. Challenges such as cost, accessibility, and the steep learning curve associated with these technologies are also analysed to provide a balanced view of the future landscape of robotic thoracic surgery.

Keywords: robotic-assisted thoracic surgery (RATS), thoracic, surgical robotics, minimally invasive surgery, mediastinum

1. Introduction

To discuss the advent of robotics in surgery we need to mention the origin of minimally invasive surgery in thoracic.

The technique of video-assisted thoracic surgery (VATS) for pulmonary lobectomy was first reported in the early 1990s. Notable contributions include Lewis RJ's discussion on "wedge resections by simultaneous stapling" and the publication "Thoracoscopic lobectomy" by Kirby TJ and Rice TW in 1993 [1, 2].

Initially, VATS was met with caution; it was recommended only for selected lobectomies and performed by thoracic surgeons who possessed advanced video-assisted surgical skills and a thorough understanding of thoracic anatomy. The innovators of VATS emphasized that it could offer a less invasive yet complete cancer operation, contrasting with the traditional more invasive approaches.

As proficiency and confidence in the technique grew, VATS lobectomy became an accepted treatment option for selected patients with stage I non-small-cell lung cancer (NSCLC) and its adoption has increased steadily [3].

During the 1980s, alongside the evolution of VATS, significant advancements in robotic technology were made to overcome the limitations of traditional VATS and laparoscopy, such as two-dimensional visualization, limited instrument mobility, and ergonomic difficulties. The advent of surgical robots transformed minimally invasive surgery by enhancing precision, flexibility, range of motion, visualization, and ergonomics. Robotic-assisted procedures maintained all the advantages of minimally invasive surgery, including less postoperative pain, smaller and cosmetically superior incisions, reduced hospital stays, and quicker recovery.

The use of robots in surgery began in 1985, initially in neurosurgery.

1.1 1985: First robotic surgery

The PUMA 560 robotic system performed the first documented use of robotics in surgery by orienting a needle for a brain biopsy under computerized tomography (CT) guidance [4].

1.2 1988: Introduction of PROBOT in urology

Developed at Imperial College London, the PROBOT was a groundbreaking advancement in medical robotics, designed specifically for urological surgery. It was utilized to autonomously perform transurethral resection of the prostate, where a three-dimensional model of the prostate was used by the robot to calculate and execute resection paths based on the surgeon's inputs. This marked a significant step towards autonomous robotic surgery [5].

1.3 1992: ROBODOC in orthopaedics

International Business Machines (IBM) and its associates developed the ROBODOC, a robotic system intended for orthopaedic surgery. This robot was primarily used to assist in accurately milling out a cavity in the femur bone during total hip replacement surgeries [6].

1.4 1994: AESOP: The robotic camera holder

The Automated Endoscopic System for Optimal Positioning (AESOP) became the first robotic device approved by the US Food and Drug Administration (FDA) for intra-abdominal surgery. Operated *via* voice commands, AESOP provided surgeons with stable, precise camera positioning, significantly enhancing surgical visibility and ergonomics. This technology laid the groundwork for later, more complex robotic surgical systems that incorporated multiple robotic arms and advanced control features.

1.5 Development of robotic telepresence technology

Robotic telepresence, developed through collaborations involving the Stanford Research Institute, the National Aeronautics and Space Administration (NASA), and the Department of Defense. Initially aimed at military applications, this technology allowed surgeons to operate remotely, using robotic arms mounted on armored vehicles for battlefield interventions. This capability expanded into civilian healthcare, providing the foundation for remote surgical procedures that connect specialists with patients across vast distances, enhancing the accessibility and efficiency of surgical care (**Figure 1**).

After acquiring the prototype, Intuitive Surgical commercialized the da Vinci Surgical System, which introduced the concept of immersive telepresence. This innovation allows surgeons to operate remotely, feeling as if they are present in the operating field, enhancing their control and reducing fatigue during procedures.

A challenge in robotic surgery is the lack of haptic feedback, which means surgeons cannot feel the tissues as they would in traditional surgery. Instead, surgeons must rely primarily on visual cues. However, recent advancements are addressing this limitation, as seen with the introduction of the latest Intuitive da Vinci model 5, which integrates enhanced sensory feedback capabilities.

While robotic systems had already gained traction in other fields, their application in thoracic surgery began with the advent of the da Vinci Surgical System by Intuitive Surgical in the early 2000s. This platform approved by the FDA in 2000 introduced the first commercially available robotic system capable of performing complex thoracic procedures with unparalleled precision.

In 2001, Melfi et al. reported the first series of robotic-assisted lobectomies. This series included five lobectomies, three tumor enucleations, three excisions, and one bulla stitching with fibrin glue for a spontaneous pneumothorax. Although three procedures required conversion to thoracotomy, all patients reported satisfactory post-operative outcomes [7].

Four years later with a larger series of 24 robotic-assisted lobectomies, they detailed specific procedural techniques, including patient positioning, port placement, and the use of surgical instruments. Two of the 24 procedures required conversion to thoracotomy [8].

In 2006, Park et al. published a retrospective case series of 34 robotic lobectomies, describing the procedures performed and the outcomes achieved. This study included

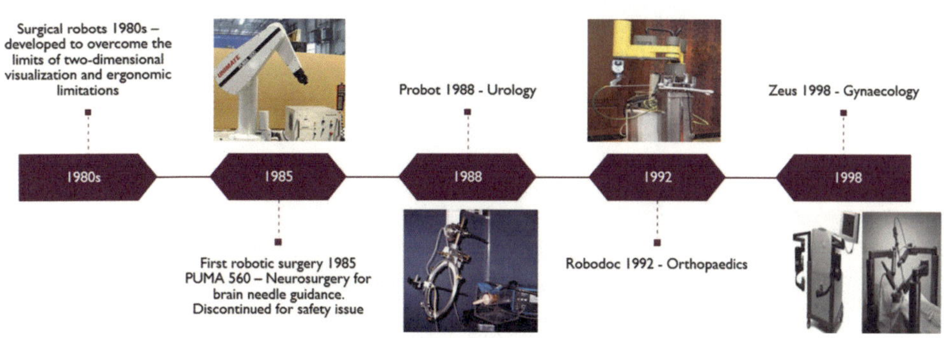

Figure 1.
Evolution of surgical robotic platforms.

a variety of lobectomy types performed on 30 patients, the majority of whom were treated for non-small-cell lung cancer. It confirmed that robotic surgery could achieve R0 resection in all cases, with four patients (12%) needing conversion to thoracotomy. The study reported no operative mortality, reinforcing the safety and effectiveness of robotic assistance in thoracic surgery [9].

The evolution of the da Vinci surgical system has brought about significant advancements, particularly with the introduction of the dual-console system in 2009. This feature has transformed the way robotic surgery is approached in terms of surgical training. The dual-console allows two surgeons to transfer control of instruments between the consoles seamlessly during a procedure. This facilitates the training of new surgeons by providing hands-on experience under direct supervision. Additionally, the telestration feature enables surgeons to annotate the operative screen in real time, marking key anatomical structures or guiding surgical movements. This functionality improves team communication during complex procedures and serves as a teaching tool for trainees, making it possible to highlight critical details without interrupting the flow of the surgery (**Figure 2**).

Another innovation is telepresence, where a surgeon operates remotely from a location separate from the operating room and the patient. An example of this technology in practice took place in Canada, where a telerobotic surgical service was established between St. Joseph's Hospital in Hamilton, Ontario, and North Bay General Hospital, located 400 kilometres away. Beginning in February 2003, this collaboration utilized a 15 Mbps IP-VPN network to connect the robotic console in Hamilton with the robotic arms of the Zeus-TS surgical system in North Bay. The network latency was reported to be between 135 and 140 milliseconds, with 14 milliseconds attributed to the distance between the two locations and the remainder due to video compression and decompression [10].

During this initiative, surgeons successfully performed 21 laparoscopic procedures remotely, including 13 fundoplication, 3 sigmoid resections, 2 right hemicolectomies,

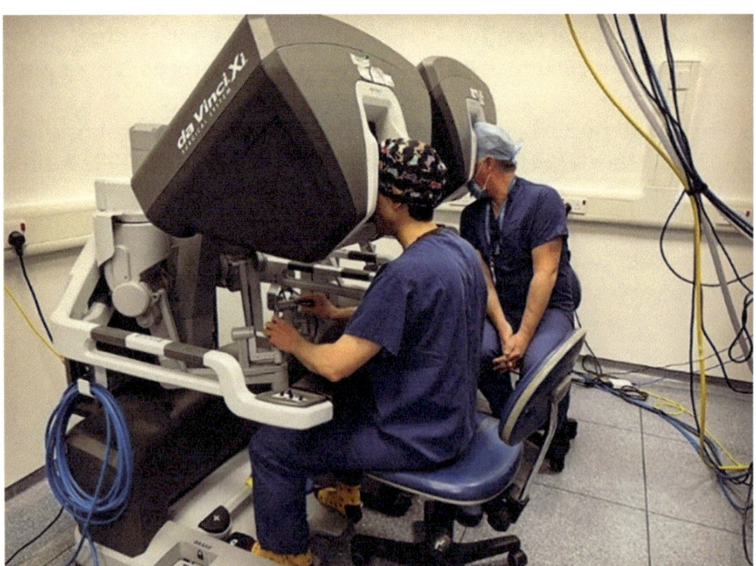

Figure 2.
Intuitive Da Vinci dual console.

1 anterior resection, and 2 inguinal hernia repairs. Despite the slight latency, the surgeons were able to adapt quickly, performing complex procedures without major intraoperative complications.

More recently in 2024 an "ultra-remote" robot-assisted right upper lobectomy between Shanghai and Kashi Prefectures was reported. A 53-year-old female from Kashi with early-stage lung cancer underwent a successful right upper lobectomy and lymph node dissection remotely controlled by surgeons in Shanghai using a dedicated 5G network. The procedure demonstrated no significant operative delays, featuring an average delay of 100 ms, and smooth postoperative recovery [11].

Additionally, telemonitoring has emerged as an essential tool in education. It allows a trainer surgeon to provide real-time mentorship to another surgeon performing a procedure, even from a remote location. This capability has significant implications for training programs, especially in regions with the limited access to specialized expertise.

2. State of the art and future perspectives

Over the last years, robotic-assisted thoracic surgery (RATS) has seen broad adoption across a wide range of thoracic procedures due to its increasing benefits. Virtually all thoracic surgery procedures benefit from the robotic approach compared to other minimally invasive approaches, such as video-assisted thoracic surgery, and certainly more so than open surgery. Evidence shows that RATS leads to fewer complications, quicker recovery, and better postoperative results. These advantages have made it a preferred method among thoracic surgeons for various surgeries, including pulmonary lobectomy, segmentectomy, resections of mediastinal masses, and esophageal surgeries.

The da Vinci surgical system is the most widely used platform for robotic thoracic surgery. It provides enhanced ergonomics and three-dimensional visualization, the da Vinci system allows for precise dissection and suturing, making it particularly advantageous for complex thoracic procedures. This platform includes four robotic arms managed from a console, providing the surgeon with stability and control that surpass traditional methods.

2.1 Components of da Vinci surgical system

Surgeon console The surgeon console is where the operating surgeon sits and controls the robotic system. It features a high-definition 3D vision system that provides a magnified view of the surgical field. The console includes master controls which the surgeon manipulates to control the robotic arms and instruments. Firefly Fluorescence Imaging integrated into the camera system can visualize blood flow and tissue perfusion using near-infrared technology. This aspect is essential in performing sublobar resections such as segmentectomies, allowing the surgeon to clearly identify the intersegmental plane.

Patient Cart The patient cart is positioned next to the operating table and holds the robotic arms and instruments. It typically includes three or four interactive robotic arms, each capable of holding various surgical instruments including the endoscopic camera (**Figures 3** and **4**).

Vision Cart acts as the hub for image processing and providing power and video for the endoscope. It also interfaces with the hospital's information systems to document and store surgical videos and data.

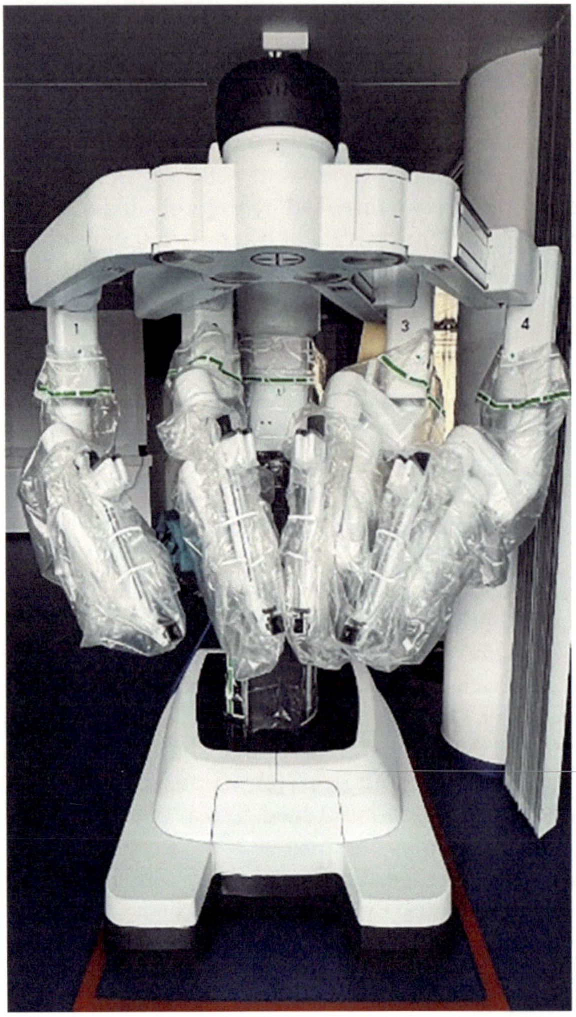

Figure 3.
Da Vinci Model Xi.

EndoWrist Instruments designed with seven degrees of freedom, a range of motion greater than the human hand. The instruments can be swapped out during surgery to suit different tasks required by the procedure (**Figure 5**).

2.2 Other platforms

The Revo-i robotic surgical system, developed by South Korean company Meerecompany and introduced in 2017, represents a cost-effective option. Designed for precise, minimally invasive procedures, the Revo-i features a master console where the surgeon's movements are translated into actions performed by robotic arms.

This system enhances surgical accuracy through its high-definition 3D visualization, which offers surgeons enhanced depth perception and magnified views. The robotic arms of the Revo-i are engineered to provide seven degrees of freedom, mirroring the dexterity and natural movements of the human wrist, thus allowing for intricate instrument manipulation within tight surgical spaces.

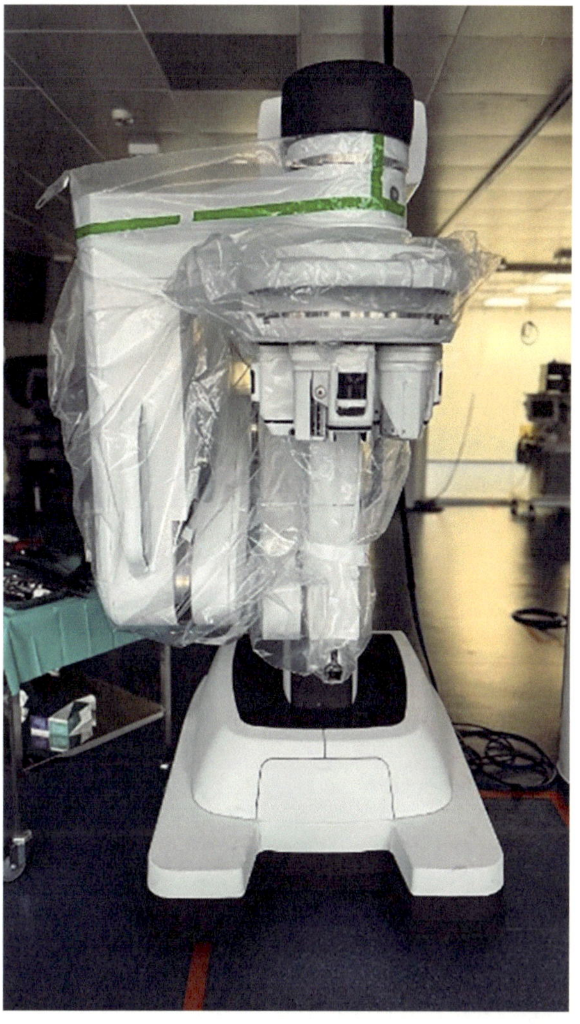

Figure 4.
Da Vinci Model SP.

One of the features of the Revo-i is its haptic feedback technology, which gives surgeons tactile sensations, akin to feeling the tissues they manipulate, thereby increasing the precision of the procedure. Additionally, its advanced optical control and camera-hopping technology afford dynamic view adjustments during surgeries, making it easier for surgeons to navigate and adapt to different surgical scenarios.

Currently, the Revo-i is employed across various surgical fields including urology, gynecology, general surgery, and thoracic surgery.

Introduced in 2019 by CMR Surgical, the Versius surgical robotic system stands out for its modular design. Each of Versius independent robotic arms can be positioned around the patient as required, providing flexibility and adaptability across various surgical environments and procedures.

Versius is engineered to support a range of surgical procedures, including those in colorectal, urological, gynecological, thoracic, and general surgeries. Its design allows surgeons to customize the setup based on the specific demands of each operation.

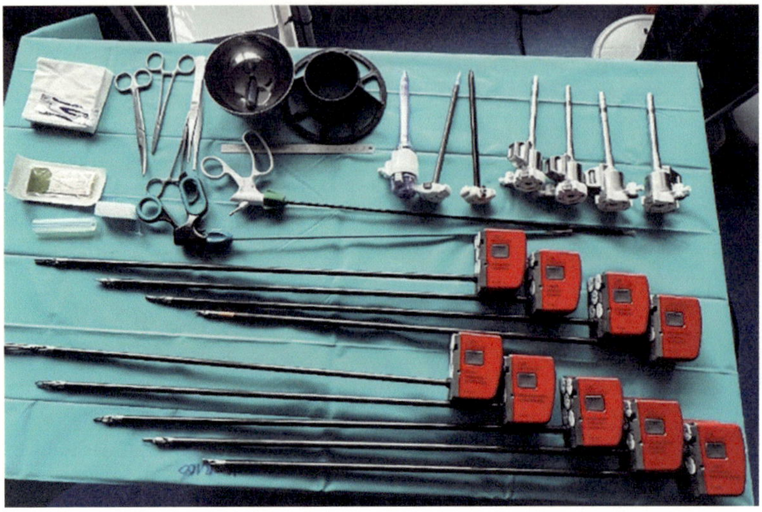

Figure 5.
EndoWrist training instruments.

Controlled *via* a surgeon console that offers a high-definition 3D view of the surgical field, Versius integrates hand-held controllers designed to replicate the natural movements of the human hand.

2.3 Robotic-assisted lung resection

Patient positioning is a critical initial step. For lung resection, patients are placed in a full lateral decubitus. The surgical table is adjusted to flex the body, with legs angled toward the floor and arms positioned in a swimmer's stance to optimize access to the thoracic cavity. Proper padding is essential to protect against nerve damage and pressure sores during the operation.

Trocar positioning, while guided by standardized protocols, often varies slightly based on the surgeon's preference and the specific requirements of the procedure. This flexibility is crucial as it allows surgeons to adapt the setup to best fit the patient's anatomy and the surgery:

- For lung resection procedures, a typical setup involves four robotic ports (two 8 mm and two 12 mm) and one 15-mm assistant port.

- The main camera port is generally placed in the 6th–7th intercostal space, slightly anterior to the scapula's tip.

- Additional ports include a 12-mm port at the anterior costal margin in the 6th–7th intercostal space and a 15-mm assistant port situated between the camera and anterior port at the 7th–8th intercostal space.

- The posterior ports are placed to enhance surgical access for the use of staplers and for retraction. 12-mm port situated one space lower than the camera port and the 8-mm port, at the edge of the paraspinal muscle, one intercostal space below the lung's major fissure.

The insertion of instruments is always carried out under direct vision to prevent damage to internal structures. Our standard instrument setup includes a Cadiere forceps, a monopolar Spatula, a robotic 3DHD camera, a SureForm robotic stapler, and a fenestrated Bipolar. For segmentectomies, the Maryland bipolar provides some advantages in the precise dissection of finer structures. Additionally, for mediastinal resections, we prefer using a Vessel Sealer to improve hemostasis in mediastinal fat (**Figures 6** and 7).

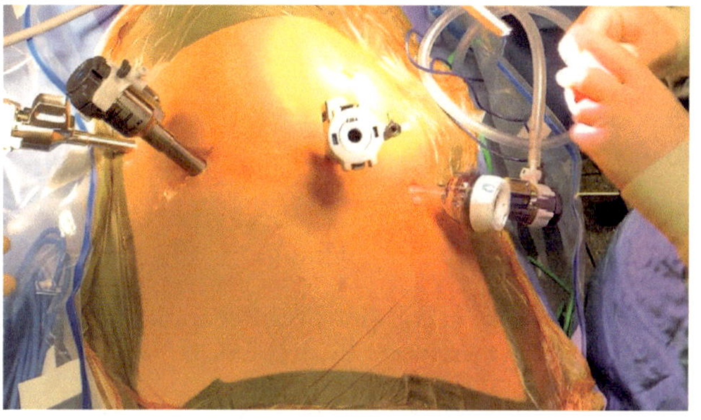

Figure 6.
Standard trocar position for lung resection. Right-side approach.

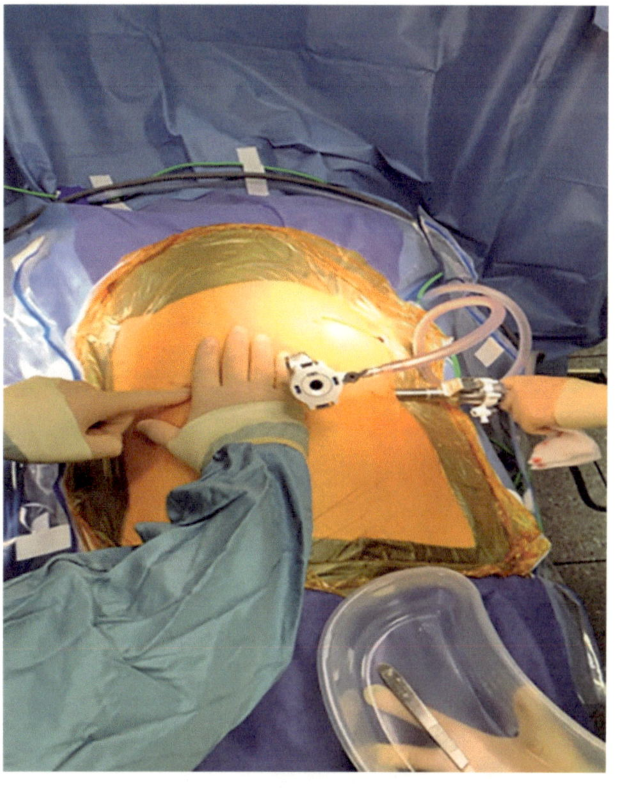

Figure 7.
Ensure trocars are positioned with adequate spacing to maximize the range of motion and clearance for the robotic arms.

Each trocar should be spaced approximately four fingers (8–10 cm) apart from each other to ensure adequate clearance for the robotic arms after docking. This setup prevents the arms clashing during the surgery (**Figure 8**).

Trocar placement is often determined by surgeon preference. For instance, the "Hamamatsu Method KAI" developed at Hamamatsu University School of Medicine using the da Vinci Xi surgical system features:

- A 30-mm access port on the posterior axillary line in the fifth intercostal space integrates an AirSeal system to maintain pneumothorax and hosts a camera, minimizing movement and enhancing stability.
- A 12-mm port positioned on the anterior axillary line in the eighth intercostal space serves as the base for the robotic stapler and acts as the second right-hand port.
- An 8-mm port, situated 8 cm caudal to the access port, accommodates robotic arm 3, controlled by the surgeon's right hand.
- Another 8-mm port, on the ventral side of the scapula in the third dorsal intercostal space, is managed by the surgeon's left hand.

This configuration minimizes the internal clash and enhances the cranial field of view.

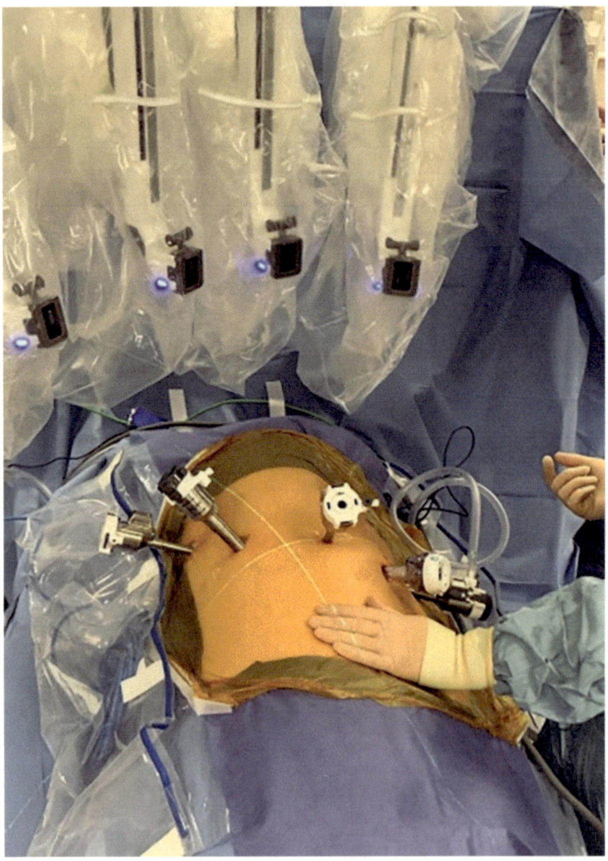

Figure 8.
Docking with target to the camera port.

2.4 Wedge resection

By reducing the extent of tissue resection, wedge resection aims to preserve lung function while achieving satisfactory oncologic outcomes in selected cases or to treat pneumothorax or perform lung volume reduction surgery. The robotic platform addresses the limitations of conventional VATS particularly in anatomically challenging areas to achieve clear margins while minimizing damage to surrounding tissue.

A study by Martin et al. compares outcomes of wedge resections for stage 1 non-small-cell lung cancer using RATS and VATS. Analyzing data from the National Cancer Database, the study included 16,559 patients from 2010 to 2019, with 80.4% undergoing VATS and 18.9% undergoing RATS. Results indicated RATS was more effective in harvesting and dissecting lymph nodes, with patients in the RATS group having a higher likelihood of lymph nodes being examined (75.2 vs. 59.0%), more nodes dissected (median of 5 vs. 4), and more frequent administration of adjuvant systemic therapy (2.2 vs. 1.3%). These findings were statistically significant even after matching based on propensity score, although nodal upstaging did not show significant difference. This suggests RATS may offer a more thorough approach in the surgical treatment of early-stage NSCLC, potentially leading to improved long-term outcomes [12].

Further supporting the advantages of robotic-assisted wedge resection, Gonzalez et al. conducted a multi-institutional review that reinforced the superiority of robotic platforms in achieving optimal lymph node harvest compared to traditional techniques [13].

In terms of technical refinements, innovative approaches such as the "lung-inverted" resection in the presence of incomplete fissure have further enhanced the feasibility of robotic-assisted wedge resections. By avoiding lung rotation in the confined thoracic cavity, this technique provides better visualization and ensure adequate surgical margins, thereby improving outcomes in anatomically challenging cases thanks to the superior visualization with the robotic camera.

A study from Pan et al. provides a detailed comparison of wedge resections performed *via* robotic-assisted thoracoscopic surgery and video-assisted thoracoscopic surgery for octogenarians with clinical stage IA non-small-cell lung cancer. It highlights that RATS significantly enhanced lymph node assessment, particularly for mediastinal lymph nodes, during wedge resections compared to VATS. In the RATS group, 57.14% of wedge resections involved mediastinal lymph node assessment versus only 16.95% in the VATS group. Again, this improved lymph node harvesting could potentially lead to better staging accuracy and tailored adjuvant therapy, additionally to the observed perioperative benefits of less bleeding and shorter hospital stays with RATS [14].

A well-known limitation of minimally invasive thoracoscopic surgery is the challenge of visualizing small lung nodules, when not subpleural, where palpation of the lesion is often not feasible. In addressing this limitation, a significant advancement has been the development of indocyanine green (ICG) dye-soaked coils for precise lung nodule localization, facilitating targeted surgical interventions. This technique was detailed in a study where ICG dye-soaked fiducial coils were used to mark pulmonary nodules prior to robotic surgeries. The method allows for accurate localization even several days after the initial placement [15].

The study, conducted on a small cohort of patients, demonstrated that the ICG dye, when soaked into fiducial coils and placed *via* robotic bronchoscopy, remained visible for up to 9 days without dispersion. This prolonged visibility is crucial for planning and executing delayed surgical resections, thus optimizing surgical outcomes, and preserving healthy lung tissue. During the robotic surgeries, the marked nodules were distinctly visible under the Firefly fluorescence imaging system of the da Vinci robotic surgery system, allowing surgeons to perform precise and minimal resections.

This technique exemplifies how robotic technologies can be synergistically combined with novel surgical aids to enhance the efficacy and safety of thoracic surgeries. It underscores the potential of robotic platforms not only to improve surgical precision but also to integrate with innovative approaches for pre-operative planning and execution.

In conclusion, emerging data suggest that robotic-assisted wedge resection holds promise in specific patient populations, particularly those with small peripheral tumors and limited respiratory reserve where minimally invasive approaches are most beneficial. Future studies should focus on multicentre prospective trials to provide robust evidence for the widespread adoption of robotic-assisted wedge resection as a standard of care and economic impact.

2.5 Segmentectomy

Segmentectomy, once mainly reserved for non-cancerous conditions such as bronchiectasis and tuberculosis, is increasingly applied in lung cancer surgeries. This transition benefits from advancements in minimally invasive techniques. The robotic approach excels in segmentectomy due to its superior precision, enhanced visualization, and greater control, which are crucial for the precise resections required in these resections. These capabilities lead to increased surgical safety and effectiveness. VATS, while valuable alternative, can be limited in complex resections by its less optimal ergonomics, restricted dissection angles, and visual access.

A retrospective study by Moon MH et al. comparing lobectomy and segmentectomy for treating early-stage non-small-cell lung cancer measuring 2 cm or less was conducted at Seoul St. Mary's Hospital, and leverages data from the SEER database spanning from 2000 to 2014, to determine whether the less invasive segmentectomy offers survival rates comparable to the more traditional lobectomy.

The study's findings challenge the conventional preference for lobectomy in certain patient demographics. The 5-year OS was 74.4% for segmentectomy and 76% for lobectomy. Hazard ratios indicated no significant difference in survival outcomes between the two surgical methods. Segmentectomy was particularly effective in elderly patients, offering a viable surgical alternative with the comparable survival outcomes. These insights suggest that segmentectomy can be a suitable alternative to lobectomy, especially for elderly patients or those with multiple comorbidities [16].

Another study by Winckelmans et al. concludes that lobectomy tends to have better survival outcomes for stage I and IA NSCLC, whereas for tumors smaller than 2 cm, segmentectomy offers comparable outcomes, providing a valuable surgical alternative especially in patients where lung preservation is crucial or when larger resections pose higher risks [17].

And more recently these results were confirmed by the CALGB 140503 (Alliance) trial compared the outcomes of lobar resection (LR), segmental resection (SR), and wedge resection (WR) in 697 patients with peripheral cT1aN0 non-small-cell lung cancer, examining disease-free survival (DFS), overall survival (OS), and lung cancer-specific survival (LCSS). Conducted between June 2007 and March 2017, the study also evaluated surgical margins, locoregional recurrence (LRR) rates, and changes in expiratory flow rate at 6-month post-operation.

Survival rates were comparable across the three methods: five-year DFS rates were 64.7% for LR, 63.8% for SR, and 62.5% for WR; OS rates were 78.7% for LR, 81.9% for SR, and 79.7% for WR; LCSS rates were 86.8% for LR, 89.2% for SR, and 89.7% for WR. There was no statistically significant difference in survival outcomes among the three groups. LRR was slightly higher in the WR group (14%) compared to the SR group (12%), but this difference was not statistically significant. Changes in forced expiratory volume (FEV1) were minimal and similar between SR and WR, showing a median reduction of 5% for WR and 3% for SR.

Overall, the study concluded that LR, SR, and WR offer similar survival benefits, with no significant differences in surgical outcomes or pulmonary function decline post-surgery [18].

The advantages of robotic platforms in performing segmentectomies have been increasingly recognized since a pivotal study by Demir et al. in 2014, which examined the outcomes in 99 patients. This research found no significant differences in morbidity and mortality when comparing robotic surgeries to traditional methods, affirming the feasibility of robotic assistance in segmentectomies [19]. Despite potentially longer operation times during the initial learning phase, the robotic approach offers superior visualization and precision. These features are particularly beneficial for complex cases requiring meticulous dissections and exacting surgical margins, making robotic systems a favored tool among thoracic surgeons for intricate procedures.

A wealth of retrospective studies and meta-analyses has reinforced the safety, feasibility, and effectiveness of robotic segmentectomy in treating lung cancer. Notably, a comprehensive study by Zhang et al. analyzed outcomes from over 45,000 patients and revealed marked benefits of robotic-assisted surgeries. These benefits encompass decreased intraoperative blood loss, lower rates of conversion to open surgery, reduced hospitalization duration, enhanced lymph node retrieval, and better 5-year disease-free survival rates, underscoring the advantages of employing robotic techniques in thoracic surgery [20].

In pulmonary segmentectomy, the segmental branches of the pulmonary arteries are traditionally divided at the fissure. However, this approach sometimes causes the pulmonary artery to be inadvertently injured and causes prolonged air leak when the fissure is incomplete.

The fissure-less technique and the lung-inverted approach are optional techniques that well fit the robotic approach. By avoiding dissection along the fissure lines, this technique minimizes the risk of bleeding and air leaks, which are common risks in lung resections.

In this approach, the surgeon accesses the lung parenchyma from the mediastinal side, moving laterally, which allows for the control of vascular and bronchial structures before they enter the lung tissue. This method is particularly advantageous in cases where the anatomy is obscured, or the fissures are poorly developed. The robotic platform enhances this technique by providing a stable and precise manipulation and superior visualization enabling more accurate dissection and staple placement without needing to manipulate the lung tissue extensively.

The lung-inverted technique is an approach in robotic surgery where the lung is manipulated to expose the posterior structures early in the procedure. This inversion is particularly useful for accessing difficult-to-reach areas or when operating on tumors located on the posterior side of the lung. It involves rotating the lung to bring the posterior section into the forefront, facilitating direct access to the target area without the need for extensive dissection through normal lung parenchyma.

This technique leverages the robotic system's ability to articulate instruments in confined spaces, allowing for precise and fine dissection around critical structures such as blood vessels and airways. The lung-inverted approach can significantly reduce operative time and enhance surgical accuracy.

Accurate dissection of intersegmental boundaries is critical in segmentectomies to ensure that the tumor is fully excised with adequate margins and without damaging it or causing ischemia in the remaining lung tissue due to improper resection sites. Traditionally, the identification of these boundaries is done by occluding the bronchi of the targeted resection zone and observing the resulting inflation-deflation line. However, this method's effectiveness is often compromised in cases with severe emphysema because the inflation-deflation line may expand *via* Kohn's alveolar pores.

Indocyanine Green, a fluorescent compound that binds to plasma proteins, offers a novel approach to delineating these intersegmental boundaries. This technique involves the resection of the primary pulmonary artery and vein in the area, followed by the intravascular administration of ICG. The lung tissue is then observed using a near-infrared camera, such as the Firefly mode on the da Vinci surgical system. This allows visualization of the lung segments that retain blood flow containing ICG, thereby providing a clear and accurate map of intersegmental boundaries based on blood flow dynamics.

2.6 Sleeve lobectomy

Pneumonectomy effectively removes lung tumors but is related to significant morbidity and mortality. Pulmonary sleeve resection is a lung-sparing surgery, primarily indicated for lung neoplasms, to preserve lung tissue by excising a lobe with the targeted lesion along with a segment of the lobar bronchus, while the bronchus serving the unaffected lobe is reconnected to the proximal airway through anastomosis. This procedure often includes bronchoplasty or vascular reconstructions.

Initially performed in the late 1940s for benign masses, it is viability for treating lung cancer was established by the mid-1950s. By the 1980s, the sleeve lobectomy became a recognized method for managing lung malignancies, particularly effective in centrally located non-small-cell lung cancer, offering superior survival and quality of life for compared to traditional pneumonectomy.

Traditionally performed with open approach, the feasibility of performing minimally invasive sleeve lobectomy was initially shown by Schmid et al. in 2011, with a combination of VATS and robotic assistance [21].

Modern robotic platforms now enable a fully robotic approach, enhancing precision and potentially improving outcomes.

Cerfolio et al. reported in 2016 a series of eight successful robotic sleeve lobectomies, with just one requiring conversion to open surgery because of intraoperative bleeding. This study underscored the capabilities of robotic systems to handle complex reconstructions, minimize surgical trauma, and improve control during operations [22].

Geraci et al. reported on a series of 23 consecutive cases undergoing sleeve resections for lung cancer, with two patients undergoing both bronchial and arterial sleeve resections (double sleeve), all managed *via* a completely robotic approach using the da Vinci Surgical System [23]. The series demonstrated very low morbidity (9%), no mortality, and a 100% rate of R0 resection, with only one case requiring conversion. The consistent success in these cases underscores the safety and efficacy of the robotic approach for this procedure, achieving comparable or superior oncologic outcomes to open approaches, with advantages including reduced postoperative pain, fewer complications, shorter hospital stays, and faster recovery.

Recent studies have illustrated the safety and feasibility of increasingly complex cases. For instance, a 74-year-old male patient with chronic obstructive pulmonary disease (COPD) presented with respiratory symptoms and was diagnosed with bilateral squamous cell carcinoma of the lungs. Given the patient's condition and the need for a conservative treatment approach, a decision was made to perform a bilateral sequential sleeve lobectomy using uniportal robotic-assisted thoracic surgery (U-RATS). This procedure was initiated with a 4-cm incision in the right seventh intercostal space. The right lower sleeve lobectomy preserved the middle lobe by anastomosing it to the bronchus intermedius using a continuous barbed suture, accompanied by a systematic nodal dissection. The patient had an uneventful recovery and was discharged on the fourth day. Subsequently, a similar procedure was carried out on the left lung; the left lower sleeve lobectomy involved the resection of the affected part of the left proximal lower bronchus. The left upper bronchus was then connected to the left main bronchus. The patient was again discharged smoothly on the 3-day post-operation [24].

A different approach for sleeve lobectomy with the same robotic platform Intuitive da Vinci performed at Shanghai Pulmonary Hospital consists only in two robotic ports (bi-portal), placed in the fourth or fifth and seventh intercostal spaces to minimize the interference between robotic arms. The use of Stratafix sutures, which are knotless barbed sutures, helped to expedite and secure the bronchial anastomosis. The study retrospectively reviewed 15 patients who underwent this procedure between March 2021 and September 2021. All patients achieved complete tumor resection without conversion to thoracotomy. The mean surgery duration was approximately 102 minutes. Average blood loss was 65 ml, and the postoperative hospital stay was around 5 days. No deaths or major complications were reported within 90-day post-surgery [25].

Sheridan et al. utilized a four-port approach to perform a sleeve right upper lobectomy with a thymic-pericardial fat flap buttress for enhanced structural support. The authors used two absorbable barbed sutures to anastomose the bronchus intermedius to the right mainstem bronchus. The thymic-pericardial fat flap was harvested and wrapped around the anastomosis site, providing additional support and protection, to reduce the risk of postoperative air leak and fistula formation [26].

Despite these advancements, challenges persist. The complex nature of robotic sleeve lobectomy, which requires significant surgical expertise and precise haptic feedback, restricts its application to highly experienced centres.

In summary, robotic sleeve lobectomy marks a significant innovation in thoracic surgery, presenting a minimally invasive but highly effective option compared to the traditional open methods. As the technique continues to evolve and become more widely adopted, it has the potential to be the preferred approach for complex airway resections.

2.7 Lobectomy

Lung lobectomy is the cornerstone treatment for operable non-small-cell lung cancer and has seen substantial advancements with the introduction of robotic-assisted thoracic surgery. Previously performed *via* open thoracotomy or VATS, the robotic platform provides significant improvements in precision, visualization, and control.

Robotic lobectomy was initially validated by early comparative research, confirming its feasibility and safety. These studies showed that it achieved oncologic outcomes similar to those of open and VATS lobectomy, and was associated with several advantages, including less blood loss, shorter hospital stays, and fewer postoperative complications [27].

Recent studies have further supported these observations, emphasizing the effectiveness of RATS in superior lymph node dissection, and enhancing long-term survival rates for early-stage non-small-cell lung cancer [28].

In 2023, the PORTal study analyzed the overall survival (OS) rates of 6646 patients undergoing robotic-assisted, video-assisted, and open lobectomy for clinical stage IA–IIIA lung cancer across 21 institutions in the United States from 2013 to 2019. To ensure adequate experience, participating surgeons were required to have performed at least 50 lobectomies before case submission. The study found that open lobectomy and robotic-assisted lobectomy were associated with higher survival rates compared to VATS, even after adjusting with propensity-score. Specifically, the unadjusted 5-year OS rates were 84% for open lobectomy, 81% for robotic-assisted, and 74% for VATS. These differences remained significant after adjustment.

The findings suggest that while minimally invasive approaches are recommended due to fewer complications and shorter hospital stays, the traditional open and robotic approach may offer better long-term survival, compared to VATS [29].

One of the main benefits of robotic lobectomy is its effectiveness in complex cases, such as those with central tumors or significant lymph node involvement. The robotic platform offers enhanced dexterity and magnified visualization, facilitating precise dissections of bronchovascular structures and lymphadenopathy. A comprehensive meta-analysis involving over 50,000 patients demonstrated that robotic lobectomy led to significantly higher rates of nodal upstaging compared to VATS, indicating a more thorough oncologic resection [30].

Beyond its clinical advantages, robotic lobectomy has driven advancements in surgical methods. The fissure-less technique, which postpones the dissection of interlobar fissures until the procedure's conclusion, has become popular for its potential to decrease air leaks and shorten operative times. Research has shown that this approach is particularly effective when utilized with robotic platforms, especially in patients with incomplete fissures [31].

2.8 Lobectomy after neoadjuvant treatment

Non-small-cell lung cancer remains one of the most prevalent cancers and a leading cause of cancer-related deaths globally. Even with curative-intent surgical resection, most patients with locally advanced disease (stages IIIA-IIIB) face high rates of distant tumor recurrence, resulting in a 5-year overall survival rate below 30%. The recent advancements in chemoimmunotherapy have transformed the treatment approach for this stage. Neoadjuvant treatments combining nivolumab and chemotherapy have demonstrated significantly improved outcomes compared to chemotherapy alone. In clinical studies, this combination yielded a longer event-free survival, with a hazard ratio for disease progression, recurrence, or death of 0.63. Furthermore, it increased the rate of pathological complete response to 24.0% versus just 2.2% with chemotherapy alone. Additional benefits were improvements in overall survival, delay in time to death or distant metastases, major pathological response, and objective response rates, as well as enhanced radiographic downstaging. Importantly, the addition of nivolumab did not elevate surgery-related complications nor affect the feasibility of surgical interventions. Patients with stage IIIA disease showed more substantial benefits from this treatment combination than those in earlier stages (IB or II) [32].

Research on neoadjuvant immunotherapy for resectable non-small-cell lung cancer includes studies like the NEOpredict-Lung trial, which explores the efficacy and safety of combined PD-1 and LAG-3 inhibitions. This trial involved NSCLC patients receiving a regimen of either Nivolumab alone or in combination with Relatlimab prior to surgical resection. A key objective was to assess the feasibility of performing surgery within 43 days after the initial treatment, a goal that was successfully achieved [33].

Although neoadjuvant therapy offers significant advantages, it is linked to hilar fibrosis and plastered tissues or inflammatory reaction leading to frail and prone to bleed tissues, which can complicate surgical procedures. Radiation can also increase the fibrosis creating indistinct dissection planes. A study by Pan and colleagues included 46 NSCLC patients who underwent immunochemotherapy prior to surgery at Shanghai Chest Hospital between 2019 and 2022. These patients were divided into two groups: 15 underwent RATS and 31 VATS.

The study observed no 30-day mortality in the RATS group and a 3.23% mortality rate in the VATS group. Patients in the RATS group experienced fewer days in intensive care and a more thorough assessment of lymph node stations compared to those in the VATS group [34].

The robotic approach has repeatedly been shown to be associated with less conversion to open when compared to VATS. The study by Feldman and colleagues evaluated 124 patients who underwent anatomic lung resection for NSCLC, with 107 receiving neoadjuvant therapy. Among these, 17 surgeries were minimally invasive, split into 9 VATS and 8 RATS. Two of the VATS procedures were non-emergently converted to open surgeries, while all robotic surgeries were completed as initially planned. The analysis revealed that patients with more than a 30% reduction in nodal short axis diameter encountered more complex surgical dissection compared to those with less than 30% reduction. cN1 disease and a nodal reduction exceeding 30% are linked to increased surgical complexity during anatomic lung resections due to nodal adherence to the pulmonary artery [35].

2.9 Lung transplantation

Lung transplantation, initially developed by pioneers like Dr. James Hardy and the Toronto Lung Transplant team, has long been the primary treatment for end-stage lung disease, historically performed through major surgical approaches. Recently, the shift towards minimally invasive techniques, including robotic-assisted surgery, has aimed to reduce complications, improving recovery, and reducing the impact on respiratory function, though widespread adoption has been gradual due to the procedure's complexity.

In February 2023, the team led by Jiao performed the first robotic-assisted lung transplant for a patient with end-stage COPD who had previously undergone bilateral pulmonary bullae resection *via* thoracotomy. This groundbreaking procedure, performed with the da Vinci Si Surgical System, involved meticulous robotic dissection to clear extensive pleural adhesions and dissect the lung hilum, removal of the right lung through an 8-cm incision. The donor lung was then inserted and robotically anastomosed. The postoperative period was smooth, with the patient being discharged on the 19th day following surgery, showing satisfactory lung expansion on follow-up imaging [36].

A few months later, in September 2023, Dr. Dominic Emerson and his team at Cedars-Sinai reported another milestone with a complete robotic-assisted lung transplant on a 69-year-old male with severe COPD. The patient's condition and anatomical considerations made him an ideal candidate. The surgery began with the robotic completion of the bronchial anastomosis and continued with the left atrial anastomosis. However, due to the prolonged ischemic time and technical difficulties with the pulmonary artery clamp, the team decided to complete the pulmonary artery anastomosis through a traditional approach, without enlarging the initial incision. The patient recovered without significant events, apart from a manageable episode of atrial fibrillation, and was discharged on the 11th postoperative day [37].

Alongside these individual case reports, Emerson's team also detailed their initial series of eight robotic lung transplants, which included a mix of single and bilateral transplants. Despite high pulmonary pressures necessitating traditional open surgical techniques in some cases, the overall outcomes were encouraging. This innovative approach not only minimized surgical invasiveness but also paved the way for potentially wider adoption of robotic assistance in lung transplants, highlighting its feasibility and benefits for patient recovery.

Other recent examples illustrate the practical application of robotic-assisted lung transplantation using typically four robotic ports and a central incision, ranging from 5 to 8 cm, for managing the graft. The surgeons tailor the placement of this incision based on personal preference and procedural necessities. As an example, Ascanio's team opts for a subxiphoid cut measuring 8 cm, Jiao's approach favors an 8-cm incision at the sixth intercostal space, while Emerson utilizes a smaller 6-cm incision at the fourth intercostal space [38, 39].

The accuracy of robotic systems significantly enhances the precision needed for complex anastomoses on bronchial, venous, and arterial structures. For bronchial anastomoses, Prolene or Polydioxanone sutures are common choices, while vascular anastomoses often require Gore-Tex or Prolene sutures. Typically, these procedures are completed without the need for extracorporeal membrane oxygenation (ECMO), though it remains an option for managing high pulmonary pressures or handling intraoperative challenges in certain cases (**Figure 9**).

New York, October 2024, in a landmark procedure, a team led by thoracic surgeons at NYU Langone Health successfully performed the world's first fully robotic double lung transplant on a 57-year-old female patient with advanced chronic obstructive pulmonary disease.

This procedure sets a new standard for lung transplant surgery and opens the door for broader application of robotic technology in complex thoracic procedures. It demonstrates the feasibility of using robotic systems for highly intricate operations that require both precision and minimal invasiveness.

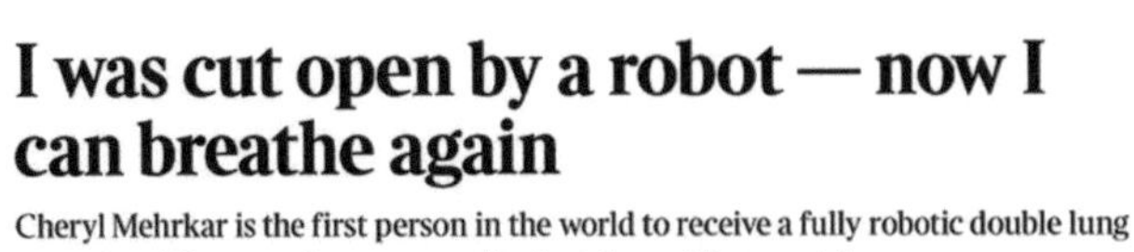
I was cut open by a robot — now I can breathe again

Cheryl Mehrkar is the first person in the world to receive a fully robotic double lung transplant. The procedure uses smaller incisions, aiding a quick recovery

Figure 9.
Title from The Times magazine, US.

While current evidence is limited to small case series, the promising results achieved indicate good potential for robotic platforms in this field.

2.10 Mediastinal mass resection and thymectomy

The robotic surgical system significantly enhances the precision and visualization in mediastinal surgeries, improving outcomes for conditions such as thymomas, substernal goiters, pericardial cysts, and neurogenic tumors like schwannomas.

Robotic surgery for mediastinal masses can be performed *via* lateral transthoracic or subxiphoid approaches, with uniport or multiport access. The choice between a subxiphoid or lateral thoracic approach largely depends on the surgeon's preference and expertise.

In a comprehensive analysis by Hong et al., 116 patients were evaluated, divided into 52 undergoing the subxiphoid approach and 64 *via* the lateral thoracic approach, all cases performed by the same surgeon. The study found that the subxiphoid approach resulted in more favorable outcomes in terms of reduced postoperative drainage, shorter drainage time, decreased postoperative hospital stays, and lower pain levels. This method appears to reduce trauma to the intercostal nerves, thus accelerating recovery, while the lateral thoracic approach registered a statistically significant shorter docking time. Both methods were safe, with no perioperative deaths, underlining the safety and feasibility of the subxiphoid approach, particularly under laryngeal mask anesthesia.

However, the analysis showed no significant differences between the two groups regarding total operative time, intraoperative bleeding, or postoperative complications.

The study does acknowledge limitations, including its retrospective design, single centre, and the lack of long-term survival data [40].

Chengwen Zheng and colleagues analyzed data from 160 cases, evenly divided between RATS and VATS. The research aimed to examine the learning curves associated with each method. The results highlighted that surgeons with VATS experience could more rapidly achieve proficiency in RATS.

Patient demographics such as age, gender, and BMI showed no notable differences between the two groups.

Operatively, both approaches demonstrated excellent patient outcomes with few complications. However, RATS recorded longer average surgery times but resulted in shorter hospital stays compared to VATS.

Analysis using the cumulative sum (CUSUM) method revealed that surgeons reached a proficiency threshold more quickly with RATS after 21 cases, as opposed to 27 cases with VATS, suggesting a more pronounced initial learning curve with VATS [41].

In their study, Qian Zheng and colleagues scrutinize the effectiveness, perioperative safety, and long-term efficacy of robotic-assisted, video-assisted, and conventional open surgery for the treatment of tumors at the mediastinal apex.

The analysis was conducted through a retrospective cohort study involving 213 patients treated from 2013 to 2023. The sample consisted of 57 RATS, 115 VATS, and 41 open cases. The findings highlighted that RATS and VATS offer significant improvements over open, in reducing intraoperative bleeding, shortening the duration of thoracic drainage, and minimizing the length of postoperative hospitalization.

RATS was particularly advantageous for managing tumors in the posterior mediastinum, better performing in this confined region. Moreover, for larger tumors exceeding 30 mm in diameter, RATS proved more effective, significantly decreasing the duration of hospital stays and effectively handling intraoperative challenges [42].

In their 2022 study published in the Journal of Thoracic Disease, Seong Yong Park and colleagues assessed the da Vinci Single-Port System (SPS) in thoracic surgeries, focusing on mediastinal mass excisions. The research evaluated the SPS's feasibility and clinical outcomes through various surgical approaches tailored to the lesions' characteristics and locations: subxiphoid, subcostal, and intercostal, used in 11, 4, and 2 cases, respectively.

The subxiphoid approach involved a single incision below the xiphoid process, allowing direct mediastinal access without xiphoid resection. The subcostal method utilized a small assistant port for CO_2 insufflation to enhance thoracic cavity access by lowering the diaphragm. The intercostal approach raised concerns about potential rib spacing and trauma.

All 17 procedures using the SPS were completed successfully without conversion to traditional multiport or open surgery, with a median operation time of 120 minutes. Patients reported minimal postoperative pain, shorter durations of *in situ* chest tube placement, and short hospital stays, indicating that the SPS could be a less invasive alternative to traditional techniques, potentially reducing recovery times and complications [43].

In their 2021 publication in the International Journal of Medical Robotics and Computer Assisted Surgery, Jia-Xin Xu and colleagues conducted a meta-analysis on a pool of 930 patients to evaluate the complications associated with robot-assisted thymectomy, comparing different surgical approaches: right-sided, left-sided, and subxiphoid.

Findings from the study indicated a lower complication rate for the left-sided approach at 7.4%, compared to 17.3% for the right-sided approach. Specific complications such as air leaks and atrial fibrillation were more prevalent in surgeries performed from the right side. Rate of pleural effusion and thoracic duct fistula did not significantly differ between approaches.

Anatomical considerations play a crucial role in selecting the surgical approach. The left-sided approach is advantageous for its enhanced visibility of critical areas, including the pericardiophrenic angle, pretracheal fatty tissue, areas behind the phrenic nerve and brachiocephalic vein, the aortopulmonary window, the aortocaval groove, anterior mediastinal fatty tissue, and the cardio phrenic angle [44].

However, many institutions often prefer a right-sided approach when the lesion's anatomical location allows. This preference is due to the greater space available for trocar positioning and reduced interference from the heart. The right-side approach also provides excellent visualization of the right phrenic nerve, superior vena cava, brachiocephalic vein, and feeding vessels for the thymus, without an increased rate of complications or anatomical procedural drawbacks.

In our practice, we position three 8-mm trocars along the margin of the major pectoralis muscle. Additionally, a 12-mm port is placed for the assistant to allow for the removal of the surgical specimen at the end of the procedure (**Figure 10**).

2.11 Robotic-assisted navigational bronchoscopy

Pulmonary nodules, commonly detected through low-dose CT scans, present a diagnostic challenge. Robotic-assisted bronchoscopy overcomes the drawbacks associated with traditional percutaneous biopsies and older bronchoscopic methods, offering a safer approach. The workflow for these robotic bronchoscopy systems

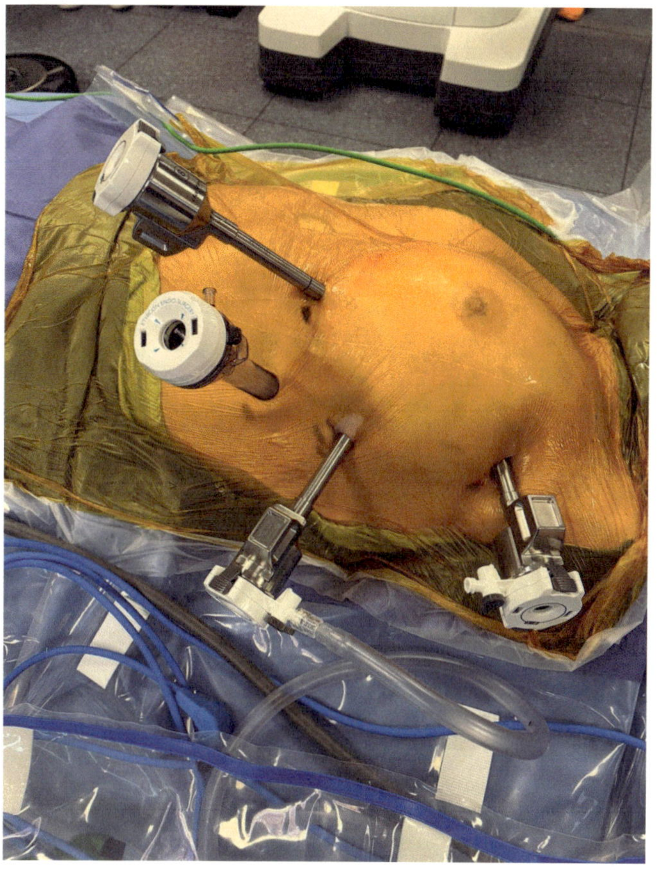

Figure 10.
Trocar position for mediastinal surgery, left-side approach.

involves detailed planning using specialized software and is typically performed under general anesthesia to maintain stable airway alignment with the planned pathway. The integration of tools such as radial endobronchial ultrasound (EBUS), fluoroscopy, and cone beam CT increases biopsy accuracy.

The FDA has approved two systems. The Monarch platform utilizes electromagnetic-navigation robotic-assisted bronchoscopy (EMN-RAB), combining a pre-procedural CT scan with electromagnetic sensors for precise targeting. This system features a console with a user-friendly interface reminiscent of a handheld gaming controller, simplifying its operation.

The Ion robotic system uses shape-sensing technology in its robotic-assisted bronchoscopy (ssRAB). It includes an internal fiber in the catheter that provides real-time positional feedback, not needing external sensors. This system has a straightforward catheter design that enhances navigability through the airways, operated by a trackball and scroll wheel for precise adjustments.

Overall, the Ion system is prized for its ease of use and adaptability, making it highly suitable for various clinical settings (not necessarily operating theater) and offering a flexible tool for pulmonary diagnostics and interventions.

A robotic bronchoscopy program requires a specialized team, including nurses, anaesthesiologists, radiology technicians, and pathologists experienced in rapid on-site evaluation (ROSE). An updated CT scan is essential, possibly 2 days before the procedure to ensure precise imaging. Optimal CT parameters should include a slice spacing of 0.5–0.8 mm for clear views of peripheral airways, a slice thickness of 0.5 mm to 1.0 mm to reduce image overlap, a minimum pitch of 1.0 to avoid motion artefacts, and a KVp of 110–140 to minimize artefacts at the lung apexes.

Coordination with the anesthesia team is important to manage patient airways effectively. Pre-operative measures to minimize secretions should include incentive spirometry and nebulizer treatments. It is advisable to use an endotracheal tube size of at least 8.5 mm, with recruitment maneuvers for prolonged intubations or in obese patients. The anticipated procedural time should be communicated to tailor the duration of paralysis, generally around 60 minutes, considering the learning curve with new programs. A minimum PEEP of 10 mm H_2O is recommended to ensure adequate ventilation of the lower lobes and reduce atelectasis risk.

Incorporating EBUS and/or cone beam CT can significantly increase biopsy precision and should be used when available. Establishing a consistent procedural protocol is paramount, including steps such as needle biopsy, brushing, transbronchial biopsy, and concluding with bronchoalveolar lavage (BAL). Ensuring enough biopsies are consistently taken and planning multiple pathways to target different lesion areas are important for comprehensive coverage and obtaining representative samples (**Figures 11(a)** and **(b)**).

A 2024 study published in *Respiration* evaluated the efficacy of shape-sensing robotic-assisted bronchoscopy versus CT-guided transthoracic biopsy (CTTB) in diagnosing subsolid pulmonary nodules, including ground-glass and part-solid types. This research was conducted retrospectively at Mayo Clinic in Florida and Rochester, spanning from February 2020 to April 2023, and involved 66 nodules from 65 patients. The findings revealed no significant difference in diagnostic yield, with ssRAB achieving 85.7% and CTTB achieving 89.5%. However, ssRAB was associated with fewer complications and facilitated mediastinal staging within the same procedure [45].

Abia-Trujillo et al., in a retrospective analysis, assessed the effectiveness of ssRAB for diagnosing ground-glass nodules and subsolid nodules with a solid component smaller than 6 mm. Conducted from September 2021 to April 2023, the research involved 22 patients and the biopsy of 23 nodules. Results indicated an 87% diagnostic yield for ssRAB, with a sensitivity for detecting malignancy at 88.9%. Adenocarcinoma was the most identified malignancy. The study also highlighted ssRAB's safety, and no complications required hospital admission or intervention [46].

A multicentre study integrating cone-beam CT with Ion Robotic Bronchoscopy, published in the *Journal of Bronchology & Interventional Pulmonology* in 2024, highlights a high diagnostic yield of 90%, with no reported pneumothorax across various centres. This indicates a significant advancement in both the efficacy and safety of this combined diagnostic approach [47].

NYU Langone Health has introduced a one-day procedure for diagnosing and surgically treating lung cancer. This method dramatically shortens the interval between diagnosis and treatment, allowing for immediate surgical intervention for early-stage lung cancer patients. Both robotic systems are utilized for diagnosis and treatment.

While pulmonologists traditionally perform bronchoscopies, thoracic surgeons bring a critical set of skills and knowledge that can greatly benefit the use of advanced systems like Ion. Thoracic surgeons are well-versed in chest anatomy and have extensive experience in managing the complexities of lung pathologies, including cancer and complications that may occur during these procedures.

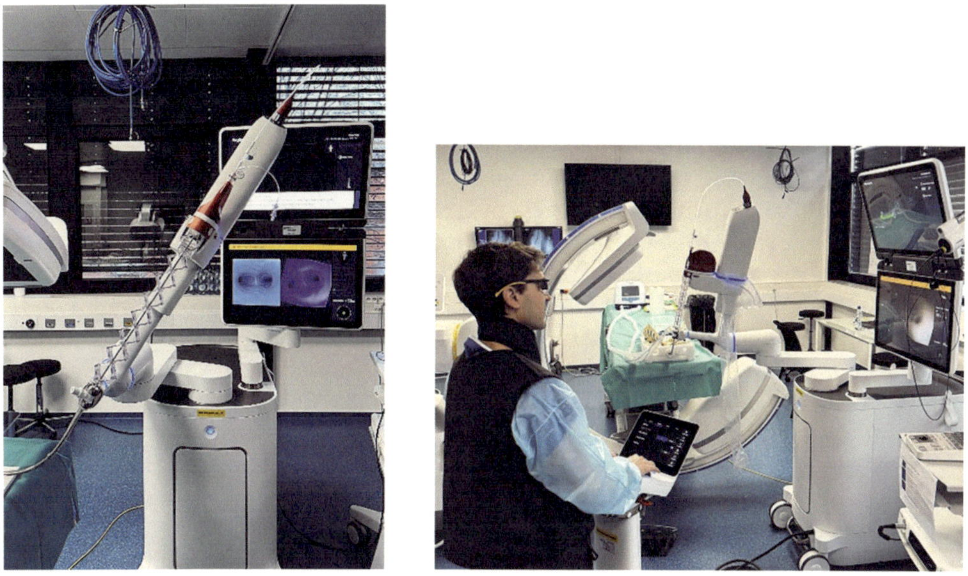

(a) (b)

Figure 11.
(a) ION robotic bronchoscopy cart and probe (training facility). (b) ION robotic bronchoscopy setup (training facility).

Surgeons are typically involved in the continuum of care from diagnosis to treatment, providing them a broader perspective that is beneficial when interpreting biopsy results and planning subsequent treatments.

2.12 Nanorobotics and AI integration

Currently, the field of nanorobotics in thoracic surgery is quite emerging and does not present extensive dedicated literature. However, the use of nanotechnology and nanorobots in medicine, including cancer treatment and other applications that could be relevant to thoracic surgery, is well-documented.

The paper titled "Nanorobotics in Medicine: A Systematic Review of Advances, Challenges, and Future Prospects with a Focus on Cell Therapy, Invasive Surgery, and Drug Delivery" explores the evolving landscape of nanorobotics and its transformative potential in biomedicine. This field merges nanotechnology with robotic capabilities to create devices that can manipulate biological systems at the nanoscale, presenting new opportunities in medical diagnostics and treatments.

Nanorobots, or nanomachines, are sophisticated mechanical or electromechanical devices engineered to perform specific tasks at a molecular level. Their size allows them to interact directly with cellular structures and biological molecules, which is particularly beneficial in medical applications such as targeted drug delivery, precision surgery, and detailed diagnostics.

In thoracic surgery, nanorobots can provide significant advantages. For instance, their ability to interact at a cellular level could revolutionize the treatment of lung cancer. Nanorobots could target cancerous cells with high precision, removing tumors with minimal damage to surrounding healthy tissues.

One part of the conventional lung cancer treatment often involves chemotherapy, which presents several side effects. Nanorobots could change this by delivering medication directly to the tumor site in the lung. This targeted approach would minimize the exposure of healthy cells to toxic chemotherapy agents, enhancing treatment efficacy and patient tolerance.

Nanorobotics has also the potential to enhance diagnostic in thoracic medicine. These tiny robots could be equipped with sensors and imaging technologies, providing real-time images and biopsies. This capability would be invaluable in early disease detection and in monitoring the progress of treatment, allowing for adjustments in real time and improving the overall management of thoracic diseases.

Despite the promising outlook, the integration of nanorobotics faces several challenges. The biocompatibility of nanorobots is a primary concern, as any foreign body can trigger an immune response in the body. Furthermore, the precise control and navigation of nanorobots within the complex internal landscape of the thoracic cavity require advanced technology and sophisticated programming to ensure accuracy and safety during operations.

Moreover, ethical and regulatory challenges must be addressed to facilitate the clinical use of nanorobots. The development of comprehensive guidelines and standards for the use of nanorobots in medicine is still necessary.

As the field of nanorobotics continues to evolve, it holds the potential to significantly alter the landscape of thoracic surgery, offering less invasive options, precise treatments, and, ultimately, better patient outcomes.

Artificial intelligence (AI) is increasingly influencing various sectors, including medicine. In medical fields such as thoracic surgery, radiology, pathology, and respiratory medicine, AI enhances patient management across all stages, from pre-operative analysis to post-operative follow-up.

However, the integration of AI into healthcare faces several challenges. A primary concern is the scarcity of data necessary for training robust AI models. Additionally, the opaque decision-making processes of AI systems complicate their validation and trust in clinical settings due to interpretability issues.

Ethical considerations are also paramount, particularly regarding privacy, consent, and the potential biases within AI algorithms that could inadvertently influence diagnostic or treatment decisions. For example, a study by Edwards et al. developed an AI algorithm that used clinical and radiological data from patients undergoing surgeries for lung nodules. This model achieved high accuracy, sensitivity, and specificity, significantly aiding in distinguishing between benign and malignant lesions, demonstrating the potential of AI to enhance diagnosis and management in thoracic surgery [48].

Deep learning has catalysed a wider adoption of AI, particularly in radiology. This technique was employed by Nam et al. [49] to identify malignant pulmonary nodules on chest radiographs. The deep learning-based algorithm not only surpassed physicians in radiograph classification and nodule detection but also significantly improved physician performance when used as a second reader.

AI has demonstrated significant potential as a tool for enhancing decision-making in thoracic surgery by providing precise assessments of surgical risks and individual prognoses for patients. Traditional risk indexes classify surgical risk based on statistical probabilities derived from large multivariate analyses that compare different population groups and the impact of various risk factors. AI, however, aims to precisely evaluate individual risk factors, allowing for tailored decision-making rather than relying on group-based risk assessments.

In a specific study, Santos-Garcia et al. [50] assessed the efficacy of an artificial neural network ensemble in predicting cardio-respiratory morbidity following pulmonary resection for non-small-cell lung cancer (NSCLC). The team trained their AI model using 348 cases and validated it with 141 cases, achieving a sensitivity of 0.67 (95% CI 0.49–0.79) and a specificity of 1.00 (95% CI 0.97–1.00). The model's area under the receiver operating characteristic curve was 0.98, indicating high predictive accuracy.

Robotic-assisted surgery is not inherently AI, though the term is often mistakenly applied in this context. With AI advancements, it is conceivable that in the future, robotic systems might autonomously perform surgeries and adapt to varying scenarios. In 2016, Shademan et al. [51] conducted a study comparing different aspects of intestinal anastomosis, including consistency of suture spacing, leakage pressure, mistakes requiring needle removal, completion time, and lumen reduction, across supervised autonomous systems (specifically the Smart Tissue Autonomous Robot, STAR), manual laparoscopic surgery, and standard robotic-assisted surgery. The STAR system demonstrated superior performance in several metrics, showing that autonomous surgery could be viable. This interaction and adaptive decision-making between the surgeon and the STAR system open new avenues for augmenting surgical procedures. Although the STAR system has successfully performed sutures in pigs, it has not yet been approved by the Food and Drug Administration for clinical use.

3. Conclusion

Robotic-assisted lung resection has proved its efficacy outpacing traditional surgery. This rise is related to the advanced technological integration within robotic platforms that support surgical precision, which minimizes intra-perioperative trauma, and reduces recovery times, benefits that are well-documented across an increasing number of studies.

When examining short-term outcomes specific to lung resection, initially, robotic-assisted thoracic surgery tends to present longer operating times when compared to VATS, an aspect linked to the initial learning curve associated with mastering robotic systems. Despite this, RATS significantly outperforms VATS by minimizing intraoperative bleeding.

In terms of complications and hospital stays, there are no significant differences between RATS and VATS. Both methods show similar rates of complications, lengths of hospital stays, and mortality rates. However, when it comes to lymph node dissection, an essential part of prognosis and treatment in cancer surgeries, RATS provides dissection of a higher number of lymph-node stations. Nevertheless, this does not necessarily translate into better oncologic staging outcomes [52].

The financial aspect of adopting RATS also plays a crucial role, particularly when viewed through the lens of the learning curve. Initially, RATS incurs higher costs primarily due to the prolonged surgical times. However, as surgical teams grow more accustomed to the robotic equipment and streamline their procedures, the duration of surgeries decreases markedly. This reduction not only aligns the operating times closer to those of VATS but also leads to a significant decrease in costs, making RATS a financially viable option over the long term [53].

On a broader scale, a prospective study conducted from July 2015 to December 2021, involving 619 patients, aimed to compare long-term oncologic outcomes such as overall survival, disease-free survival, and recurrence rates between RATS and VATS. Robotic-assisted surgeries showed a statistically significant improvement in disease-free survival and a lower recurrence rate, suggesting a potential advantage in managing cancer more effectively [54].

Moreover, when focusing on the quality-of-life changes from pre- to post-surgery, utilizing the European Organization for Research and Treatment of Cancer (EORTC) quality of life questionnaires, RATS patients demonstrated notable improvements. They experienced considerably lower postoperative symptoms such as dyspnoea, fatigue, and pain compared to those who underwent VATS or thoracotomy [55].

In conclusion, although robotic-assisted thoracic surgery (RATS) presents initial challenges such as longer operation times and higher start-up costs, the long-term benefits in patient outcomes and overall cost savings make a strong case for its adoption.

Conflict of interest

The authors declare no conflict of interest.

Author details

Alessandro Maraschi[1*], Thomas Fraccalini[2] and Kunal Bhakhri[1]

1 University College London Hospital, Thoracic Surgery, London, United Kingdom

2 Department of Medical and Oncology, Division of Geriatrics Medicine, San Luigi Gonzaga Hospital, Turin, Italy

*Address all correspondence to: alessandro.maraschi@gmail.com

IntechOpen

© 2025 The Author(s). Licensee IntechOpen. This chapter is distributed under the terms of the Creative Commons Attribution License (http://creativecommons.org/licenses/by/4.0), which permits unrestricted use, distribution, and reproduction in any medium, provided the original work is properly cited.

References

[1] Lewis RJ. The role of video-assisted thoracic surgery for carcinoma of the lung: Wedge resection to lobectomy by simultaneous individual stapling. The Annals of Thoracic Surgery. 1993;**56**:762-768

[2] Kirby T, Rice T. Thoracoscopic lobectomy. The Annals of Thoracic Surgery. 1993;**56**:784-786

[3] McKenna RJ, Wolf RK, Brenner M, et al. Is lobectomy by videoassisted thoracic surgery an adequate cancer operation? The Annals of Thoracic Surgery. 1998;**66**:1903-1908

[4] Kwoh YS, Hou J, Jonckheere EA, Hayati S. A robot with improved absolute positioning accuracy for CT guided stereotactic brain surgery. IEEE Transactions on Biomedical Engineering. 1988;**35**:153-160

[5] Davies BL, Hibberd RD, Coptcoat MJ, Wickham JEA. A surgeon robot prostatectomy—A laboratory evaluation. Journal of Medical Engineering & Technology. 1989;**13**:273-277

[6] Bauer A, Borner M, Lahmer A. Clinical experience with a medical robotic system for total hip replacement. In: Nolte LP, Ganz R, editors. Computer Assisted Orthopedic Surgery. Bern: Hogrefe & Huber; 1999. pp. 128-133

[7] Melfi FM, Menconi GF, Mariani AM, et al. Early experience with robotic technology for thoracoscopic surgery. European Journal of Cardiothoracic Surgery. 2002;**21**(5):864-868

[8] Melfi FM, Ambrogi MC, Lucchi M, Mussi A. Video robotic lobectomy. Multimedia Manual of Cardio-thoracic Surgery. 1 Jan 2005;**2005**(628): mmcts.2004.000448. DOI: 10.1510/mmcts.2004.000448. PMID: 24414727

[9] Park BJ, Flores RM, Rusch VW. Robotic assistance for video assisted thoracic surgical lobectomy: Technique and initial results. The Journal of Thoracic and Cardiovascular Surgery. 2006;**131**(1):54-59

[10] Anvari M, McKinley C, Stein H. Establishment of the world's first telerobotic remote surgical service: For provision of advanced laparoscopic surgery in a rural community. Annals of Surgery. 2005;**241**:460-464

[11] Tian Y, Lv H, Jumai A, Tuerhong T, Zhuang L, Huang J, et al. Ultra-remote robot-assisted right upper lobectomy between the Shanghai and Kashi prefectures: A case report. Journal of Thoracic Disease. 31 Dec 2024;**16**(12):8823-8830. DOI: 10.21037/jtd-24-1605. Epub 2024 Dec 27. PMID: 39831214; PMCID: PMC11740061

[12] Martin J et al. Outcomes of robotic vs video-assisted Thoracoscopic wedge resections: A propensity-matched analysis using National Cancer Database Data. Journal of Thoracic Oncology. 2020;**15**(4):763-772. DOI: 10.1016/j.jtho.2019.10.011

[13] Gonzalez M et al. Advantages of robotic thoracic surgery in achieving optimal lymph node harvest: A multi-institutional review. Annals of Thoracic Surgery. 2021;**112**(2):392-398. DOI: 10.1016/j.athoracsur.2020.10.032

[14] Pan H, Zou N, Tian Y, Shen Y, Chen H, Zhu H, et al. Robotic versus thoracoscopic sub-lobar resection for octogenarians with clinical stage IA

non-small cell lung cancer: A propensity score-matched real-world study. Annals of Surgical Oncology. 2024;**31**(3):1568-1580. DOI: 10.1245/s10434-023-14689-5 Epub 2023 Dec 10

[15] Bawaadam H, Benn BS, Colwell EM, Oka T, Krishna G. Lung nodule marking with ICG dye–soaked coil facilitates localization and delayed surgical resection. Annals of Thoracic Surgery Short Reports. 2023;**1**(2):221-225. DOI: 10.1016/j.atssr.2023.02.010. ISSN 2772-9931

[16] Moon MH, Moon YK, Moon SW. Segmentectomy versus lobectomy in early non-small cell lung cancer of 2 cm or less in size: A population-based study. Respirology. 2018;**23**(7):695-703. DOI: 10.1111/resp.13277. Epub 2018 Feb 21

[17] Winckelmans T, Decaluwé H, De Leyn P, Van Raemdonck D. Segmentectomy or lobectomy for early-stage non-small-cell lung cancer: A systematic review and meta-analysis. European Journal of Cardio-Thoracic Surgery. 2020;**57**(6):1051-1060. DOI: 10.1093/ejcts/ezz339

[18] Altorki N, Wang X, Damman B, Mentlick J, Landreneau R, Wigle D, et al. Lobectomy, segmentectomy, or wedge resection for peripheral clinical T1aN0 non–small cell lung cancer: A post hoc analysis of CALGB 140503 (Alliance). The Journal of Thoracic and Cardiovascular Surgery. 2024;**167**(1):338-347.e1. DOI: 10.1016/j.jtcvs.2023.07.008. ISSN 0022-5223

[19] Demir A et al. Morbidity and mortality in robotic vs non-robotic segmentectomy: A prospective analysis of 99 patients. Thoracic Surgery Clinics. 2014;**24**(4):385-395. DOI: 10.1016/j.thorsurg.2014.05.003

[20] Zhang X et al. Outcomes of robotic-assisted segmentectomy: A comprehensive analysis of over 45,000 cases. Lung Cancer. 2020;**149**:110-120. DOI: 10.1016/j.lungcan.2020.10.007

[21] Schmid T, Augustin F, Kainz G, Pratschke J, Bodner J. Hybrid video-assisted thoracic surgery-robotic minimally invasive right upper lobe sleeve lobectomy. The Annals of Thoracic Surgery. Jun 2011;**91**(6):1961-1965. DOI: 10.1016/j.athoracsur.2010.08.079. PMID: 21619991

[22] Cerfolio RJ et al. Robotic sleeve lobectomy: Case series of eight patients with successful outcomes. Journal of Thoracic and Cardiovascular Surgery. 2016;**152**(1):64-70. DOI: 10.1016/j.jtcvs.2016.01.040

[23] Geraci TC, Ferrari-Light D, Wang S, et al. Robotic sleeve resection of the airway: Outcomes and technical conduct using video vignettes. The Annals of Thoracic Surgery. 2020;**110**:236-240. DOI: 10.1016/j.athoracsur.2020.01.077

[24] Gonzalez-Rivas D, Prado RF, Garcia-Perez A, Bosinceanu ML, Motas N, Manolache V. Bilateral uniportal robotic-assisted thoracic surgery sleeve lobectomy for a bilateral endobronchial lung cancer. Annals of Cardiothoracic Surgery. 2023;**12**(1):64-66. DOI: 10.21037/acs-2022-urats-10. Epub 2022 Dec 20

[25] Qu JC, Zhang WT, Jiang L. Two-port robotic sleeve lobectomy using Stratafix sutures for central lung tumors. Thoracic Cancer. 2022;**13**(10):1457-1462. DOI: 10.1111/1759-7714.14412. Epub 2022 Apr 6

[26] Sheridan B, Zhao J, Jung C, Doño A, Koffman E, Valaulikar G, et al. Robotic sleeve right upper lobectomy with thymic/pericardial fat flap buttress. JTCVS Techniques. 2024;**28**:164-167. DOI: 10.1016/j.xjtc.2024.09.009

[27] Melfi FM et al. Robotic lobectomy for lung cancer: Early results and challenges. Journal of Thoracic and Cardiovascular Surgery. 2018;**156**(3):930-937. DOI: 10.1016/j.jtcvs.2018.02.045

[28] Yang CF et al. Comparative outcomes of robotic-assisted, video-assisted, and open lobectomy for early-stage non-small cell lung cancer: A meta-analysis. Journal of Thoracic Oncology. 2022;**17**(2):222-232. DOI: 10.1016/j.jtho.2021.11.007

[29] Kent MS, Hartwig MG, Vallières E, Abbas AE, Cerfolio RJ, Dylewski MR, et al. Pulmonary open, robotic, and thoracoscopic lobectomy (PORTaL) study: Survival analysis of 6646 cases. Annals of Surgery. 2023;**277**(6):1002-1009. DOI: 10.1097/SLA.0000000000005820

[30] Cerfolio RJ et al. The fissureless technique in robotic lobectomy: Reducing air leaks and optimizing outcomes. Innovations in Thoracic Surgery. 2019;**15**(3):187-193. DOI: 10.1177/1753466619838723

[31] Gonzalez-Rivas D et al. Uniportal robotic lobectomy: A minimally invasive technique for the future. European Journal of Cardiothoracic Surgery. 2020;**58**(3):590-598. DOI: 10.1093/ejcts/ezz099

[32] Forde PM, Spicer J, Lu S, et al. Neoadjuvant Nivolumab plus chemotherapy in resectable lung cancer. The New England Journal of Medicine. 2022;**386**:1973-1985

[33] Shields MD, Lovly CM. Refining neoadjuvant immunotherapy for resectable lung cancer. Nature Medicine. 2024;**30**:1535-1536. DOI: 10.1038/s41591-024-03001-x

[34] Pan H, Zou N, Tian Y, et al. Short-term outcomes of robot-assisted versus video-assisted thoracoscopic surgery for non-small cell lung cancer patients with neoadjuvant immunochemotherapy: A single-center retrospective study. Frontiers in Immunology. 2023;**14**:1228451

[35] Feldman HA, Zhou N, Deboever N, et al. Intraoperative challenges after induction therapy for non-small cell lung cancer: Effect of nodal disease on technical complexity. JTCVS Open. 2022;**12**:372-384

[36] Jiao W, Yang R, Zhao Y, Ge N, Qiu T, Sun X, et al. Robot-assisted single lung transplantation. Chinese Medical Journal. 2023;**136**(3):362-364. DOI: 10.1097/CM9.0000000000002462

[37] Emerson D, Catarino P, Rampolla R, Chikwe J, Megna D. Robotic-assisted lung transplantation: First in man. The Journal of Heart and Lung Transplantation. 2024;**43**(1):158-161

[38] Ascanio L et al. Robotic-assisted lung transplantation using a subxiphoid approach: A case series. Journal of Thoracic and Cardiovascular Surgery. 2022;**164**(3):789-797. DOI: 10.1016/j.jtcvs.2022.05.012

[39] Jiao W et al. Minimally invasive lung transplantation: Insights from robotic-assisted techniques. European Journal of Cardiothoracic Surgery. 2023;**65**(1):44-52. DOI: 10.1093/ejcts/ezac098

[40] Hong Z, Sheng Y, Bai X, et al. Clinical efficacy of robot-assisted subxiphoid versus lateral thoracic approach in the treatment of anterior mediastinal tumors. World Journal of Surgical Oncology. 2023;**21**:94

[41] Zheng C, Ge Y, Ma T, Pan J, Zhang X, Sun T, et al. Outcomes of robot-assisted versus video-assisted

mediastinal mass resection during the initial learning curve. Journal of Robotic Surgery. 2024;**18**(1):81. DOI: 10.1007/s11701-024-01828-7

[42] Zheng Q, Ma YF, Jiang SS, Yu-Wen S, Xu Y, Liu Y. Comparison of three methods in the surgical treatment of mediastinal roof tumors. Journal of Thoracic Disease. 2024;**16**(10):6368-6380. DOI: 10.21037/jtd-24-946. Epub 2024 Oct 30

[43] Park SY, Lee JH, Stein H, et al. Initial experience with and surgical outcomes of da Vinci single-port system in general thoracic surgery. Journal of Thoracic Disease. 2022;**14**:1933-1940

[44] Xu JX, Qian K, Deng Y, Zheng YY, Ou CM, Liu J, et al. Complications of robot-assisted thymectomy: A single-arm meta-analysis and systematic review. The International Journal of Medical Robotics. 2021;**17**(6):e2333. DOI: 10.1002/rcs.2333. Epub 2021 Sep 24

[45] Fernandez-Bussy S, Yu Lee-Mateus A, Reisenauer J, Balasubramanian P, Barrios-Ruiz A, Garza-Salas A, et al. Shape-sensing robotic-assisted bronchoscopy versus computed tomography-guided transthoracic biopsy for the evaluation of subsolid pulmonary nodules. Respiration. 2024;**103**(5):280-288. DOI: 10.1159/000538132. Epub 2024 Mar 12

[46] Abia-Trujillo D, Chandra NC, Koratala A, Yu Lee-Mateus A, Garza-Salas A, Barrios-Ruiz A, et al. Diagnostic yield of shape-sensing robotic-assisted bronchoscopy for ground-glass nodules and subsolid nodules with a solid component less than 6 mm. Respiration. 2023;**102**(10):899-904. DOI: 10.1159/000533314. Epub 2023 Aug 24

[47] Reihani AR, Zohouri M, Thomas J. Breaking new ground in interventional pulmonology: Integrating cone beam CT and robotic-assisted bronchoscopy for high-risk pneumothorax in peripherally located solitary pulmonary nodules. Cureus. 2024;**16**(6):e62532. DOI: 10.7759/cureus.62532

[48] Edwards FH, Schaefer PS, Cohen AJ, et al. Use of artificial intelligence for the preoperative diagnosis of pulmonary lesions. The Annals of Thoracic Surgery. 1989;**48**:556-559

[49] Nam JG, Park S, Hwang EJ, et al. Development and validation of deep learning-based automatic detection algorithm for malignant pulmonary nodules on chest radiographs. Radiology. 2019;**290**:218-228

[50] Santos-Garcia G, Varela G, Novoa N, et al. Prediction of postoperative morbidity after lung resection using an artificial neural network ensemble. Artificial Intelligence in Medicine. 2004;**30**:61-69

[51] Shademan A, Decker RS, Opfermann JD, et al. Supervised autonomous robotic soft tissue surgery. Science Translational Medicine. 2016;**8**:337ra364

[52] Lampridis S, Maraschi A, Le Reun C, Routledge T, Billè A. Robotic versus video-assisted thoracic surgery for lung cancer: Short-term outcomes of a propensity matched analysis. Cancers. 2023;**15**(8):2391. DOI: 10.3390/cancers15082391

[53] Harrison OJ, Maraschi A, Routledge T, Lampridis S. A cost analysis of robotic vs. video-assisted thoracic surgery: The impact of the learning curve and the COVID-19 pandemic. Frontiers in Surgery. 2023;**10**:1123329. DOI: 10.3389/fsurg.2023.1123329

[54] Fabbri G, Femia F, Lampridis S, Farinelli E, Maraschi A, Routledge T, et al. Long-term oncologic outcomes in robot-assisted and video-assisted lobectomies for non-small cell lung cancer. Journal of Clinical Medicine. 2023;**12**(19):6230. DOI: 10.3390/jcm12196230

[55] Asemota N, Maraschi A, Lampridis S, Pilling J, King J, Le Reun C, et al. Comparison of quality of life after robotic, video-assisted, and open surgery for lung cancer. Journal of Clinical Medicine. 2023;**12**(19):6230. DOI: 10.3390/jcm12196230

Chapter 2

Surgical Procedures

Mustafa Karaağaç

Abstract

Gastroesophageal reflux disease (GERD) is a chronic condition characterized by the backflow of stomach contents into the esophagus, affecting millions of people worldwide. Its pathophysiology involves a combination of factors, including the weakening of the lower esophageal sphincter (LES), increased intra-abdominal pressure, delayed gastric emptying, and hiatal hernia. Although lifestyle modifications and pharmacological treatments are usually sufficient to control symptoms, some patients may require surgical intervention when these approaches are inadequate. The goals of surgical treatment for GERD include anatomical correction, elimination of reflux symptoms, and prevention of complications. Surgical indications include symptoms resistant to medical therapy, dependence on and side effects of medications, reflux-related complications, and hiatal hernia. This chapter provides a detailed examination of the indications for surgical treatment of GERD, the surgical techniques used, and the advantages, disadvantages, and potential complications of these techniques.

Keywords: gastroesophageal reflux disease, minimally invasive surgery, surgical indications in gastroesophageal reflux, hiatal hernia, transoral incisionless fundoplication

1. Introduction

Gastroesophageal reflux disease (GERD) is a chronic condition characterized by the backflow of stomach contents into the esophagus, typically presenting with symptoms such as heartburn, regurgitation, and chest pain [1]. GERD is a prevalent health issue affecting millions of people worldwide and can significantly reduce the quality of life [2]. The pathophysiology of the disease can involve a combination of factors, including the weakening of the lower esophageal sphincter (LES), increased intra-abdominal pressure, delayed gastric emptying, and hiatal hernia [3]. While lifestyle modifications and pharmacological treatments may be sufficient for most patients, these approaches may be inadequate or result in long-term side effects for some individuals. Specifically, surgical intervention may become necessary for patients who do not respond to medication, develop medication dependency, or experience complications [4].

The goals of surgical treatment for gastroesophageal reflux disease include anatomical correction, elimination of reflux symptoms, and prevention of complications [5]. This chapter will comprehensively examine the indications for surgical treatment of GERD, the surgical techniques utilized, and the advantages, disadvantages, and potential complications of these techniques.

2. Indications for surgical treatment of gastroesophageal reflux disease

2.1 Symptoms resistant to medical therapy

A significant portion of GERD patients can control their symptoms with acid-suppressive medications such as proton pump inhibitors (PPIs) and H2 receptor antagonists [6]. However, patients whose symptoms remain uncontrolled despite these medications may be candidates for surgical intervention. Medically resistant GERD can significantly reduce the patient's quality of life, and surgical treatment may offer an effective solution for symptom relief and improvement in quality of life [7].

2.2 Medication dependency and side effects

For patients requiring long-term use of PPIs and H2 receptor antagonists, the side effects and costs of these medications can be significant concerns. Long-term use of PPIs can lead to various side effects, including decreased absorption of vitamins and minerals, kidney disease, osteoporosis, and an increased risk of infections [8]. Therefore, surgical treatment may be a suitable option for patients who do not wish to continue medication indefinitely or want to avoid the long-term side effects of these medications.

2.3 Reflux-related complications

Severe complications of GERD are among the most critical indications for surgical treatment. These complications include Barrett's esophagus, a condition where the cells in the lower part of the esophagus undergo abnormal changes due to chronic reflux. Barrett's esophagus is a significant risk factor for the development of esophageal adenocarcinoma, and patients with this condition may be evaluated for surgical treatment to reduce the risk of cancer development [9]. Another complication, esophagitis, involves inflammation and erosion of the esophageal mucosa. This common complication of chronic reflux can lead to ulcers and strictures in the esophagus, and severe cases of esophagitis may require surgical intervention [9]. Strictures, or narrowing of the esophagus, can cause swallowing difficulties and are considered a serious complication. Surgical treatment may be necessary to correct these narrowings in patients with strictures [9]. Additionally, aspiration pneumonia, infections resulting from stomach contents entering the lungs, is a significant risk, particularly in patients with nocturnal reflux. In patients with recurrent aspiration pneumonia, surgical intervention can help control reflux and prevent lung complications [10].

2.4 Hiatal hernia

Hiatal hernia is characterized by the protrusion of a portion of the stomach through the esophageal hiatus of the diaphragm into the chest cavity. This anatomical alteration can exacerbate gastroesophageal reflux symptoms and worsen the severity of the disease [11]. Hiatal hernias are anatomically classified into four types: Type I (sliding), Type II (paraesophageal), and Type III (mixed); Type IV hiatal hernia is a large and complex paraesophageal hernia in which, in addition to the stomach, other intra-abdominal organs (e.g., colon or spleen) also migrate through the diaphragmatic hiatus into the thoracic cavity. The sliding type is the most common and is often associated with reflux. In this type of hernia, the gastroesophageal junction moves above the diaphragm, causing the stomach to herniate. In paraesophageal hiatal hernia, the gastroesophageal junction remains in place while a portion of the stomach herniates beside the esophagus into the chest cavity. The mixed type involves features of both sliding and paraesophageal hernias.

The contribution of hiatal hernia to reflux can be explained through several mechanisms. Firstly, hiatal hernia reduces the pressure of the LES, preventing its effective closure and allowing gastric contents to reflux into the esophagus. Secondly, in the presence of hiatal hernia, the crural muscles of the diaphragm cannot support the LES, increasing reflux episodes. Thirdly, the abnormal positioning of the stomach fundus in hiatal hernia facilitates the backflow of stomach acid and food into the esophagus.

In sliding hiatal hernia, the LES moves above the diaphragm, reducing its effectiveness and leading to reflux. Postprandial increases in intra-abdominal pressure can further impair the LES function, facilitating the backflow of gastric contents into the esophagus. This mechanism can result in more frequent and severe reflux symptoms.

In paraesophageal hiatal hernia, although the LES remains in place, a portion of the stomach herniates into the chest beside the esophagus. This abnormal positioning of the stomach fundus can still facilitate the backflow of gastric contents and acid into the esophagus, leading to reflux symptoms even if the LES function is preserved. In mixed type hiatal hernias, both sliding and paraesophageal features are present, resulting in more complex and severe reflux symptoms.

Understanding the relationship between hiatal hernia and reflux is crucial for treatment planning. Repairing hiatal hernia plays a significant role in reducing reflux symptoms by supporting the LES and restoring normal anatomical structure. During hiatal hernia repair, the surgeon reduces the size of the diaphragmatic hiatus and reinforces the tissues around the esophagus by suturing them. This aims to reposition the stomach back into the abdominal cavity and restore normal anatomical configuration.

Postoperative outcomes typically include a significant reduction in reflux symptoms and improved quality of life for patients [11]. However, individual patient characteristics and risk factors must be carefully evaluated when deciding on surgical treatment. The risks of postoperative complications, the patient's overall health status, and the surgeon's experience should also be considered. Patient education about the surgical procedure and postoperative care is critical for treatment success. Informing patients about the surgical procedure and closely monitoring them in the postoperative period is essential for the early detection and management of complications.

Type I hiatal hernias can generally be managed with medical therapy. Reflux symptoms can be controlled with medications such as proton pump inhibitors or H2 receptor antagonists. However, in patients who do not respond to medical treatment or develop severe complications, surgical intervention is necessary. In these cases, Nissen fundoplication is often the preferred method [11]. This procedure, performed laparoscopically, involves wrapping the fundus of the stomach around the esophagus to prevent reflux. This approach is minimally invasive, allowing for faster patient recovery and reduced postoperative pain. Type II hiatal hernias typically require surgical intervention due to the risk of strangulation and potential severe complications. Regardless of symptoms, paraesophageal hernias necessitate surgical repair. These interventions are usually performed using open or laparoscopic techniques and involve steps such as hernia sac removal, hiatus narrowing, and fundoplication. The laparoscopic approach is less invasive, promoting faster postoperative recovery. During surgery, various techniques are employed to ensure the esophagus remains in the anatomically correct position. Type III hiatal hernias often necessitate surgical intervention due to the risks of strangulation and volvulus [11]. In these cases, laparoscopic or open hiatal repair and fundoplication are the preferred surgical options. Laparoscopic surgery is frequently chosen for its minimally invasive nature and the quicker postoperative recovery it offers. Surgical intervention includes hernia repair, repositioning the stomach to its anatomical position, and performing a fundoplication. These steps help control reflux symptoms and reduce the risk of hernia recurrence. The patient's overall health status and other comorbidities must be carefully assessed during surgical planning. Type IV hiatal hernias generally require surgical intervention. Due to the serious symptoms and complications these hernias can cause, emergency surgery may be necessary. Surgical repair of Type IV hernias can be complex, involving the removal of the hernia sac, narrowing of the hiatus, and repositioning of the displaced organs to their anatomical locations. The laparoscopic approach is preferred for its minimally invasive nature, reduced postoperative pain, and faster recovery time. The patient's overall health status and other comorbidities must be carefully evaluated. Additionally, when multiple organs are displaced, more extensive surgical intervention may be required.

2.5 Patient preference and quality of life

Some patients may prefer surgical intervention over continuous medication use. Surgical treatment can offer a long-term solution compared to medical therapy and significantly enhance patients' quality of life [12]. Patient preferences, lifestyle, and suitability for surgery play a crucial role in determining surgical indications. Compared to medical treatment, surgical therapy can provide faster and more permanent symptom control.

2.6 Young patients and long-term treatment planning

Patients diagnosed with GERD at a young age and requiring lifelong medical therapy may be directed towards surgical treatment to avoid the long-term side effects of medication. For these patients, surgical intervention can be a more sustainable treatment option. Achieving symptom relief through a surgical solution rather than lifelong medication can be advantageous in terms of long-term health outcomes for young patients.

2.7 GERD associated with obstructive sleep apnea

Patients with obstructive sleep apnea (OSA) frequently exhibit GERD, which can further deteriorate sleep quality [13]. GERD can exacerbate OSA and lead to more frequent apneic episodes during sleep. Controlling GERD through surgical intervention can help alleviate OSA symptoms [13]. In these patients, reflux surgery aims to improve sleep quality and overall health.

2.8 Atypical symptoms associated with reflux

In addition to typical symptoms, GERD can present with atypical manifestations, including chronic cough, laryngitis, asthma-like symptoms, and chest pain [14].

Atypical symptoms that do not respond to medical therapy may require surgical intervention. Surgical treatment can be effective in alleviating these symptoms, particularly in patients with persistent atypical symptoms despite PPI therapy.

2.9 Reflux confirmed by functional tests

When deciding on surgical intervention, it is important to confirm the diagnosis of GERD through functional tests. Tests such as pH monitoring, esophageal manometry, and impedance-pH monitoring play a critical role in confirming the diagnosis of reflux and determining surgical indications [15]. These tests help identify patients who are suitable candidates for the surgical treatment of GERD.

3. Preoperative evaluation in patients with GERD

3.1 Detailed patient history and symptom analysis

A comprehensive patient history forms the first step in preoperative evaluation. This process involves determining the duration of the patient's symptoms and the extent to which these symptoms affect daily life and functionality. Specific triggers, such as postprandial or nocturnal heartburn, should be investigated. The type of symptoms should also be carefully assessed, including the frequency, duration, and intensity of heartburn felt in the chest area; the occurrence and frequency of regurgitation; the character and duration of chest pain; differentiation from cardiac causes; and the stage at which dysphagia symptoms arise. Additionally, the presence of atypical symptoms such as chronic cough, hoarseness, laryngitis, and asthma-like symptoms, and their response to medical therapy should be reviewed [16].

The patient's response to previous medical treatments and the effectiveness of these treatments in controlling symptoms are also crucial aspects of the evaluation. The results obtained with proton pump inhibitors (PPIs) and H2 receptor antagonists should be particularly noted. The impact of lifestyle and dietary changes on symptoms should also be assessed. For example, have measures like elevating the head of the bed, avoiding certain foods, and weight loss alleviated symptoms? The answers to these questions are critical in treatment planning.

3.2 Imaging and functional tests

Before planning surgical treatment, a series of imaging and functional tests should be conducted to confirm the diagnosis of GERD and examine anatomical details. Upper gastrointestinal endoscopy provides a direct visual assessment of the esophagus, stomach, and duodenum. Endoscopy is crucial for detecting complications such as erosive esophagitis, Barrett's esophagus, strictures, and hiatal hernia [17]. Additionally, biopsies can be taken for histopathological examination.

The 24-hour pH monitoring, which measures the amount of acid reflux in the esophagus, is the gold standard for confirming the diagnosis of GERD [18]. This test determines the correlation between the patient's symptoms and acid reflux episodes, providing critical data for surgical decision-making [18]. Esophageal manometry evaluates the motor function of the esophagus and the pressure of the LES. Manometry identifies esophageal motility disorders and is critical for surgical planning [19]. Poor esophageal peristalsis can influence the choice of surgical technique.

A barium swallow radiograph is an imaging method using barium contrast to examine the anatomical structure and function of the esophagus. This method is effective in demonstrating hiatal hernias, strictures, and other structural anomalies, particularly in identifying conditions like paraesophageal hernias that may require surgery. Impedance-pH monitoring detects both acidic and nonacidic reflux events, especially used in patients unresponsive to PPI therapy. Impedance-pH monitoring plays a significant role in treatment planning by identifying the acidic or non-acidic nature of reflux.

These evaluations and tests are of great importance for the accurate identification of GERD and determining appropriate treatment methods. This comprehensive evaluation process before surgical intervention ensures the correct management of patients' symptoms and increases the success rate of treatment.

4. Transoral incisionless fundoplication with or without hiatal hernia repair in gastroesophageal reflux disease

Transoral Incisionless Fundoplication (TIF) is an advanced endoscopic procedure used in the treatment of GERD and is considered a minimally invasive method. TIF can be performed with or without hiatal hernia repair and aims to alleviate the reflux symptoms in patients [20]. During the TIF procedure, general anesthesia is administered to the patient, who is positioned supine. An endoscope is inserted through the mouth and advanced towards the esophagus, and the EsophyX device, specifically designed for TIF, is attached to the endoscope. This device is advanced into the stomach to reach the gastroesophageal junction. The first step of the procedure involves cleaning and preparing the gastroesophageal junction area. Subsequently, using the EsophyX device, the fundus of the stomach is pulled upwards, creating a fold between the esophagus and the stomach. This fold acts as a barrier against reflux, preventing gastric acid from regurgitating into the esophagus.

In the TIF procedure, special fasteners are used to secure the fundoplication. Typically, between 10 and 20 fasteners are placed, creating approximately a 270° fundoplication. At this stage, the integrity of the fundoplication and the correct placement of the fasteners are endoscopically verified.

The complications of the TIF procedure can include both acute and long-term issues. Acute complications encompass risks such as bleeding, perforation, and infection. Bleeding can occur during or after the procedure and is usually controlled by endoscopic methods. Perforation involves the creation of a hole in the esophageal or gastric wall due to the use of the endoscope or the EsophyX device, which may necessitate emergency surgical intervention. The risk of infection, as with any surgical procedure, is present and can generally be mitigated with prophylactic antibiotic use.

Short- and long-term complications include dysphagia, complaints of gas and bloating, and the persistence of reflux symptoms. Dysphagia is characterized by difficulty swallowing due to narrowing of the esophageal opening, which is often temporary. Some patients may experience gas and bloating complaints due to the entry of air into the stomach and the fundoplication. Additionally, in cases where a hiatal hernia is present, GERD symptoms may not completely resolve or may recur. In instances where symptoms persist due to insufficient fundoplication, a repeat TIF procedure or alternative surgical interventions may be necessary.

TIF offers an effective option in the treatment of GERD due to its minimally invasive nature and rapid recovery process [20]. However, patient selection, preoperative evaluation, and management of potential complications are critical to the procedure's success. Detailed patient assessment and the identification of appropriate indications are paramount for the efficacy and safety of the TIF procedure. Individual risks and benefits should be evaluated for each patient to determine the most suitable treatment approach. TIF plays a significant role in GERD treatment due to its less invasive nature and shorter recovery period compared to traditional surgical methods [20].

5. Magnetic sphincter strengthening

Magnetic sphincter augmentation (MSA) is an innovative minimally invasive surgical method used in the treatment of GERD. The primary goal of MSA is to strengthen the weakened LES to prevent the backflow of stomach contents into the esophagus. This procedure involves the placement of a ring composed of magnetic beads around the LES, aiming to alleviate GERD symptoms [21]. The procedure is performed under general anesthesia and employs laparoscopic surgical techniques.

Before initiating the MSA procedure, a thorough evaluation of the patient is conducted. This evaluation includes tests such as endoscopy, pH monitoring, and manometry to confirm the diagnosis of GERD. During the procedure, the patient is positioned supine and general anesthesia is administered. The surgeon makes five small incisions in the abdominal area, which are necessary for the insertion of laparoscopic instruments and the camera into the abdominal cavity.

After gaining access to the abdominal cavity, CO_2 gas is used to inflate the cavity. The surgeon carefully dissects the fat tissue and other structures around the stomach and esophagus to reach the lower part of the esophagus. Once the lower esophagus is fully exposed, the MSA device, consisting of magnetic beads, is placed around the esophagus. The MSA device is a ring made of titanium-coated beads, each containing a magnetic core. These beads exert a continuous pressure around the esophagus, reinforcing the LES.

After the MSA device is placed around the esophagus, the beads are magnetically attracted to each other. This magnetic attraction ensures the closure of the LES, preventing gastric acid from refluxing into the esophagus. During swallowing, the beads separate to allow the passage of food into the stomach. Once swallowing is completed, the beads reattach, ensuring the closure of the LES. This dynamic movement allows for the normal functioning of the swallowing and digestive processes.

Post-MSA, patients typically experience a rapid recovery, with most returning to normal activities within a few days. However, due to the nature of the surgical procedure, some complications may arise. Complications of the MSA procedure include both acute and chronic issues. Acute complications include bleeding, infection, and perforation. Bleeding may occur during or after the procedure and can be controlled laparoscopically if necessary. The risk of infection, as with any surgical procedure, exists and can be reduced with prophylactic antibiotic use. Perforation is a rare but serious complication that requires emergency surgical intervention. Early detection and management of these complications positively influence the patient's recovery process.

Long-term complications include dysphagia, device migration or erosion, and the persistence of reflux symptoms. Dysphagia can occur due to the inability of the magnetic ring around the esophagus to expand during swallowing and is usually temporary. However, in some cases, dysphagia may be persistent and require additional intervention. Device migration or erosion is a rare but serious complication, potentially necessitating surgical removal of the device. The persistence or recurrence of reflux symptoms may indicate insufficient efficacy of MSA, warranting additional treatment approaches.

The success of the MSA procedure depends on appropriate patient selection and correct surgical technique. Detailed patient assessment and the identification of proper indications are crucial for the efficacy and safety of the MSA procedure. MSA provides a significant option in GERD treatment due to its minimally invasive nature and rapid recovery process. However, like any surgical procedure, potential complications and risks must be carefully considered. MSA plays a significant role in GERD treatment due to its less invasive nature and shorter recovery period compared to traditional surgical methods. The most suitable treatment approach should be determined by evaluating individual risks and benefits for each patient.

Studies on the long-term efficacy and safety of MSA demonstrate its success in alleviating GERD symptoms and improving patients' quality of life [22]. However, due to the novelty of this procedure, further research is needed to understand its long-term outcomes and potential complications. When applied with appropriate indications and by experienced surgeons, MSA offers an effective and safe option for GERD treatment. Therefore, evaluating and implementing the MSA procedure for suitable candidates can be a significant step in GERD treatment [22].

6. Partial fundoplications

6.1 Dor fundoplication

Dor fundoplication is a partial fundoplication technique used in the surgical treatment of GERD. This technique involves wrapping the LES 180°. The aim is to strengthen the LES to prevent the backflow of stomach contents into the esophagus [23]. Dor fundoplication is typically performed laparoscopically, facilitating faster recovery with a minimally invasive approach.

The Dor fundoplication procedure begins under general anesthesia, with the patient positioned supine. The surgeon makes five small incisions in the abdominal area to allow for the insertion of laparoscopic instruments and the camera into the abdominal cavity. The surgeon frees the gastric fundus and reaches the lower part of the esophagus. The gastric fundus is wrapped 180° around the esophagus to create a barrier around the LES. This wrap strengthens the LES and prevents gastric acid from refluxing into the esophagus. In Dor fundoplication, the anterior wall of the fundus is wrapped around the right and left sides of the esophagus and sutured. This technique involves wrapping the anterior wall without releasing the structures behind the LES. The fundus is anchored to the anterior wall of the esophagus, thereby strengthening the LES. During the procedure, care is taken to avoid damaging the surrounding tissues of the esophagus and stomach while freeing and wrapping the fundus.

The recovery process after Dor fundoplication is typically quick due to the use of minimally invasive techniques, allowing patients to return to normal activities within a few days.

Complications of Dor fundoplication include bleeding, infection, perforation, dysphagia, and gas complaints. Bleeding may occur during or after the procedure and can be controlled laparoscopically if necessary. The risk of infection exists, as with any surgical procedure, and can be reduced with prophylactic antibiotic use. Perforation involves damage to the esophageal or gastric wall, requiring emergency surgical intervention. Dysphagia, usually temporary, manifests as difficulty

DOI: http://dx.doi.org/10.5772/intechopen.1006670

swallowing post-fundoplication. Gas complaints can arise due to air entering the stomach and difficulties in releasing gas. These complications can be managed with surgical intervention and postoperative care.

6.2 Toupet fundoplication

Toupet fundoplication is another partial fundoplication technique used in the treatment of GERD. This technique involves wrapping the LES 270° to prevent the backflow of stomach acid into the esophagus [24]. Toupet fundoplication is preferred when a complete wrap around the LES is not appropriate and may be more suitable for patients with motility disorders [24].

The Toupet fundoplication procedure begins under general anesthesia, with the patient positioned supine. Five small incisions are made in the abdominal area to allow for the insertion of laparoscopic instruments and the camera into the abdominal cavity. CO_2 gas is used to inflate the abdominal cavity, facilitating the visualization of the surgical field. The surgeon frees the gastric fundus and reaches the lower part of the esophagus. In Toupet fundoplication, the gastric fundus is wrapped 270° around the back of the esophagus (**Figure 1**). This creates a broader wrap around the LES, reducing reflux symptoms. The fundus is sutured to the posterior wall of the esophagus and wrapped on both sides.

The advantage of Toupet fundoplication is that it supports the LES without completely encircling it [24]. This can reduce the risk of dysphagia and may be more suitable for patients with motility disorders. Proper wrapping and suturing of the fundus strengthen the LES and prevent gastric acid from refluxing into the esophagus. Care is taken during the procedure to avoid damaging surrounding tissues while freeing and wrapping the fundus.

The recovery process after Toupet fundoplication is typically quick due to the use of minimally invasive techniques, allowing patients to return to normal activities within a few days.

Complications of Toupet fundoplication include bleeding, infection, perforation, dysphagia, and gas complaints [24]. Bleeding may occur during or after the procedure and can be controlled laparoscopically if necessary. The risk of infection exists, as with any surgical procedure, and can be reduced with prophylactic antibiotic use.

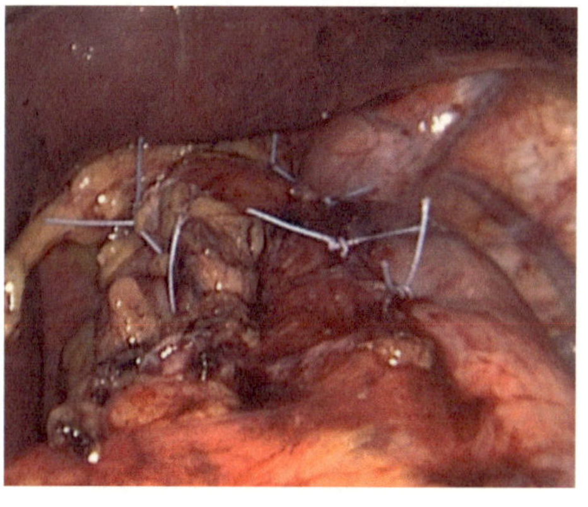

Figure 1.
In toupet repair, the stomach fundus is released by passing it through the posterior part of the abdominal esophagus and suturing it to the right and left of the esophagus in such a way that it surrounds the esophagus at 270°.

Perforation involves damage to the esophageal or gastric wall, requiring emergency surgical intervention. Dysphagia, usually temporary, manifests as difficulty swallowing post-fundoplication. Gas complaints can arise due to air entering the stomach and difficulties in releasing gas. These complications can be managed with surgical intervention and postoperative care.

Both fundoplication methods can be effective in the treatment of GERD, but patient selection and the appropriate use of techniques are critical for the success of the procedure and the prevention of complications. Dor and Toupet fundoplications offer significant options in GERD treatment due to their minimally invasive nature and rapid recovery times. However, potential complications and risks should be carefully considered, as with any surgical procedure. Individual risks and benefits should be evaluated for each patient to determine the most appropriate treatment approach. Studies on the long-term efficacy and safety of Dor and Toupet fundoplications have shown these methods to be successful in alleviating GERD symptoms and improving patients' quality of life [24]. However, more research is needed on the long-term outcomes and potential complications of these procedures. When performed with the correct indications and by experienced surgeons, Dor and Toupet fundoplications offer effective and safe options in GERD treatment.

7. Nissen fundoplication

Nissen fundoplication is one of the most commonly used surgical treatments for GERD [25]. This procedure aims to prevent the backflow of stomach contents into the esophagus by creating a 360° wrap around the LES. Nissen fundoplication is typically performed laparoscopically, although open surgery may be required in some cases. When performed using a minimally invasive approach, the recovery time is faster, and postoperative pain is less.

The Nissen fundoplication procedure begins under general anesthesia, with the patient positioned supine. The surgeon makes five small incisions in the abdominal area for the insertion of laparoscopic instruments and the camera into the abdominal cavity. Following the first incision, CO_2 gas is introduced into the abdominal cavity with the help of a trocar.

The surgeon starts by freeing the gastric fundus. During this process, the short gastric vessels are cut and dissected. These vessels are released to separate the gastric fundus from the spleen and surrounding tissues. This step ensures that the fundus is of sufficient length and flexibility to form a complete wrap around the LES.

Once the lower part of the esophagus is fully exposed, any hiatal hernia present is repaired. During hiatal hernia repair, the hiatus opening in the diaphragm is reduced, and the tissues around the esophagus are sutured to secure it. This ensures a tighter junction between the stomach and esophagus, preventing the backflow of stomach contents. Hiatal hernia repair is a critical step for the success of the fundoplication and must be performed carefully by the surgeon [25].

The primary step of Nissen fundoplication is wrapping the gastric fundus 360° around the esophagus (**Figure 2**). The surgeon wraps the fundus around the esophagus and sutures the ends of the fundus together to secure it. This wrap creates a cuff around the LES, supporting its closure. The complete wrap of the gastric fundus prevents the backflow of stomach acid into the esophagus, thereby reducing GERD symptoms. During the wrapping process, care is taken to ensure that the lower part of the esophagus remains free and mobile to preserve natural movements during swallowing.

DOI: http://dx.doi.org/10.5772/intechopen.1006670

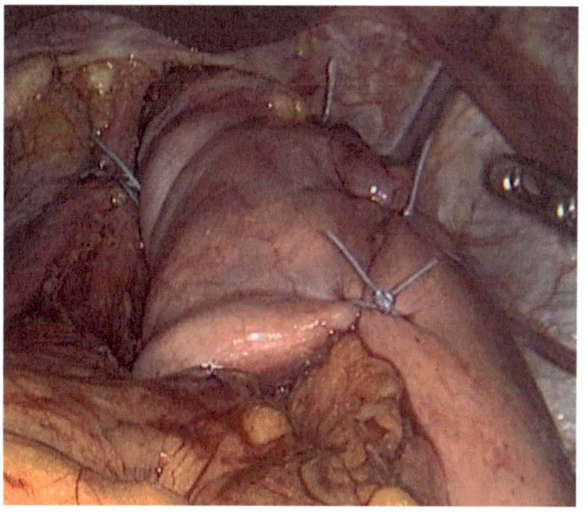

Figure 2.
In the Nissen repair, the stomach fundus is released by passing it through the posterior abdominal esophagus and sutured to surround the esophagus 360°, and the hiatus defect is sutured.

Proper positioning and tension of the fundus wrap are crucial for the success of the procedure. Wrapping the fundus too tightly increases the risk of dysphagia; therefore, the tension of the wrap is carefully adjusted during the procedure.

The recovery process after Nissen fundoplication is typically quick due to the use of minimally invasive techniques, allowing patients to return to normal activities within a few days.

Complications of Nissen fundoplication include bleeding, infection, perforation, dysphagia, and gas complaints. Bleeding may occur during or after the procedure and can be controlled laparoscopically if necessary. The risk of infection exists, as with any surgical procedure, and can be reduced with prophylactic antibiotic use. Perforation involves damage to the esophageal or gastric wall, requiring emergency surgical intervention. Dysphagia, usually temporary, manifests as difficulty swallowing post-fundoplication. This can occur due to a too-tight wrap of the fundus or restricted esophageal mobility. Gas complaints arise due to air entering the stomach and difficulties in releasing gas, leading to bloating and discomfort after meals. Some patients may experience difficulties with belching and vomiting post-Nissen fundoplication.

Long-term complications of Nissen fundoplication include loosening or unraveling of the wrap, recurrence of hiatal hernia, and persistence of reflux symptoms. Loosening or unraveling of the wrap can result in the loss of the cuff effect around the LES, leading to the recurrence of reflux symptoms [25]. Recurrence of hiatal hernia occurs when the gastric fundus slips through the diaphragm again, potentially necessitating additional surgical intervention. Persistent or recurrent reflux symptoms may occur when the fundoplication is inadequate, requiring alternative treatment methods for these patients.

Nissen fundoplication is an effective method for treating GERD, but patient selection and the use of appropriate surgical techniques are critical for the success of the procedure and the prevention of complications. Laparoscopic Nissen fundoplication offers a significant option in GERD treatment due to its minimally invasive nature and rapid recovery time. However, potential complications and risks should be carefully evaluated, as with any surgical procedure. Studies on the long-term efficacy and safety of Nissen fundoplication have shown this method to be successful in alleviating GERD symptoms and improving patients' quality of life [25]. Nevertheless, more research is needed on the long-term outcomes and potential complications of this procedure. Nissen fundoplication, when performed with the correct indications and by experienced surgeons, offers an effective and safe option in GERD treatment.

Individual risks and benefits should be evaluated for each patient to determine the most appropriate treatment approach. Nissen fundoplication remains an important option for patients seeking a permanent solution for GERD. However, as with any surgical procedure, patient education and postoperative care are critical to treatment success. Informing patients about the surgical procedure and closely monitoring them in the postoperative period are essential for early detection and management of complications. The effectiveness and safety of Nissen fundoplication can be ensured through proper patient selection, correct application of surgical techniques, and postoperative care [25].

8. Conclusion

The management of GERD has significantly evolved with advancements in both diagnostic and therapeutic modalities. The selection of appropriate treatment strategies, whether medical or surgical, is contingent upon a thorough understanding of the pathophysiology, precise patient evaluation, and the application of individualized treatment plans. Minimally invasive surgical options such as MSA and TIF offer promising outcomes for selected patients, enhancing quality of life with reduced recovery times and lower complication rates. However, ongoing research is imperative to fully elucidate the long-term efficacy and safety of these interventions. A multidisciplinary approach, encompassing patient education, careful preoperative assessment, and vigilant postoperative monitoring, is essential to optimize treatment outcomes and ensure patient safety in the management of GERD.

Acknowledgements

We are grateful to Prof. Dr. Muhammet Akyüz of the Department of General Surgery, Faculty of Medicine, Erciyes University, for providing the images.

The author acknowledges the use of ChatGPT for language polishing of the manuscript.

Conflict of interest

The authors declare no conflict of interest.

DOI: http://dx.doi.org/10.5772/intechopen.1006670

Author details

Mustafa Karaağaç
General Surgery, Erciyes University Faculty of Medicine, Kayseri, Turkey

*Address all correspondence to: drmustafakaraagac@gmail.com

IntechOpen

© 2024 The Author(s). Licensee IntechOpen. This chapter is distributed under the terms of the Creative Commons Attribution License (http://creativecommons.org/licenses/by/4.0), which permits unrestricted use, distribution, and reproduction in any medium, provided the original work is properly cited.

References

[1] Chhabra P, Ingole N. Gastroesophageal reflux disease (GERD): Highlighting diagnosis, treatment, and lifestyle changes. Cureus. 2022;**14**(8):e28563

[2] Nirwan JS, Hasan SS, Babar ZUD, Conway BR, Ghori MU. Global prevalence and risk factors of gastro-oesophageal reflux disease (GORD): Systematic review with meta-analysis. Scientific Reports. 2020;**10**(1):5814

[3] Fuchs KH, Lee AM, Breithaupt W, Varga G, Babic B, Horgan S. Pathophysiology of gastroesophageal reflux disease—Which factors are important? Translational Gastroenterology and Hepatology. 2021;**6**:53

[4] Antunes C, Aleem A, Curtis SA. Gastroesophageal Reflux Disease. Treasure Island, FL: StatPearls Publishing; 2017

[5] Lopes SO, Gonçalves AR, Macedo G, Santos-Antunes J. Endoscopic treatment of gastroesophageal reflux: A narrative review. Porto Biomedical Journal. 2023;**8**(4):e226

[6] Kröner PT, Cortés P, Lukens FJ. The medical management of gastroesophageal reflux disease: A narrative review. Journal of Primary Care and Community Health. 2021;**12**:21501327211046736

[7] Naik RD, Meyers MH, Vaezi MF. Treatment of refractory gastroesophageal reflux disease. Gastroenterology and Hepatology. 2020;**16**(4):196

[8] Maideen NMP. Adverse effects associated with long-term use of proton pump inhibitors. Chonnam Medical Journal. 2023;**59**(2):115

[9] Warners MJ, Nijhuis RAO, de Wijkerslooth LR, Smout AJ, Bredenoord AJ. The natural course of eosinophilic esophagitis and long-term consequences of undiagnosed disease in a large cohort. Official Journal of the American College of Gastroenterology|ACG. 2018;**113**(6):836-844

[10] Pisegna J, Holtmann G, Howden CW, Katelaris PH, Sharma P, Spechler S, et al. Oesophageal complications and consequences of persistent gastro-oesophageal reflux disease. Alimentary Pharmacology and Therapeutics. 2004;**20**:47-56

[11] Sfara A, Dumitrascu DL. The management of hiatal hernia: An update on diagnosis and treatment. Medicine and Pharmacy Reports. 2019;**92**(4):321

[12] Kendrick K, Kothari SN. Updates on surgical treatment for gastroesophageal reflux disease. The American Surgeon™. 2023;**89**(6):2730-2737

[13] Mahfouz R, Barchuk A, Obeidat AE, Mansour MM, Hernandez D, Darweesh M, et al. The relationship between obstructive sleep apnea (OSA) and gastroesophageal reflux disease (GERD) in inpatient settings: A nationwide study. Cureus. 2022;**14**(3):e22810

[14] Wu J, Ma Y, Chen Y. GERD-related chronic cough: Possible mechanism, diagnosis and treatment. Frontiers in Physiology. 2022;**13**:1005404

[15] Vardar R, Keskin M. Indications of 24-h esophageal pH monitoring, capsule pH monitoring, combined pH monitoring with multichannel impedance, esophageal manometry,

radiology and scintigraphy in gastroesophageal reflux disease. The Turkish Journal of Gastroenterology. 2017;**28**(Suppl. 1):S16-S21

[16] Campbell KA, Madva EN, Villegas AC, Beale EE, Beach SR, Wasfy JH, et al. Non-cardiac chest pain: A review for the consultation-liaison psychiatrist. Psychosomatics. 2017;**58**(3):252-265

[17] Asreah RH, Abdullhameed A. Risk factors of erosive esophagitis and barrett's esophagus in patients with reflux symptoms. Medical Journal of the Islamic Republic of Iran. 2021;**35**:75

[18] Marabotto E, Savarino V, Ghisa M, Frazzoni M, Ribolsi M, Barberio B, et al. Advancements in the use of 24-hour impedance-pH monitoring for GERD diagnosis. Current Opinion in Pharmacology. 2022;**65**:102264

[19] Pham T, Telias I, Beitler JR. Esophageal manometry. Respiratory Care. 2020;**65**(6):772-792

[20] Bomman S, Malashanka S, Ghafoor A, Sanders DJ, Irani S, Kozarek RA, et al. Safe implementation of transoral incisionless fundoplication as a new technique in a tertiary care center. Clinical Endoscopy. 2022;**55**(5):630-636

[21] Patel A, Gyawali CP. The role of magnetic sphincter augmentation in the gastroesophageal reflux disease treatment pathway: The gastroenterology perspective. Diseases of the Esophagus. 2023;**36**(Suppl. 1):doad 005

[22] Sarici IS, Dunn CP, Eriksson SE, Jobe BA, Ayazi S. Long-term clinical and functional results of magnetic sphincter augmentation. Diseases of the Esophagus. 2023;**36**(Suppl. 1):doac109

[23] Loo GH, Rajan R, Tata MD, Kosai NR. Changes in the disease-specific quality of life following dor fundoplication. A multicentre cross-sectional study. Annals of Medicine and Surgery. 2020;**55**:252-255

[24] Gunter RL, Shada AL, Funk LM, Wang X, Greenberg JA, Lidor AO. Long-term quality of life outcomes following Nissen versus Toupet fundoplication in patients with gastroesophageal reflux disease. Journal of Laparoendoscopic and Advanced Surgical Techniques. 2017;**27**(9):931-936

[25] Seeras K, Bittar K, Siccardi MA. Nissen Fundoplication. In: StatPearls [Internet]. Treasure Island, FL: StatPearls Publishing; Jan 2024. PMID: 30137806

Section 2

Orthopedic Surgery

Chapter 3

Pediatric Fractures Treated by Resorbable Implants

Gergo Jozsa and Marcell Varga

Abstract

Biodegradable implants have seen an increase in application in pediatrics. Designed to naturally dissolve over time, they offer a promising alternative to traditional metal implants by reducing long-term complications. Initially limited to fixation of knee joint fractures—where the need for a material that could safely degrade as the bone heals was first recognized—since then, their application has expanded considerably. Today, these are effectively employed to treat fractures in the ankle and elbow joints. More recently, the use of these implants has extended to fractures in the forearm and wrist, further demonstrating their versatility and growing acceptance in pediatric orthopedics. The study provides a comprehensive overview of the indications for implants—from clavicle to ankle—and details the surgical techniques required for proper fixation. Illustrations are also offered for visual evidence of successful outcomes. A major advantage is their ability to offer results comparable to metal counterparts. Despite being newer, resorbable implants have proven equally effective and safe over the years. Their ability to dissolve naturally renders them a viable option for pediatric patients, minimizing the need for future surgical interventions. This process reduces the risk of infections, complications of removal, or foreign material reactions. In summary, resorbable implants represent an important advancement in the treatment of childhood fractures. Their expanding range of applications, from the clavicle to the ankle, along with the positive clinical outcomes associated with their use, positions them as a highly effective and less invasive alternative to traditional metal implants in pediatric fracture management.

Keywords: children, resorbable implants, forearm fractures, ankle fractures, osteochondral fractures of the knee, elbow fractures

1. Introduction

The use of resorbable implants, especially in the treatment of childhood fractures, is currently not one of the primary procedures of choice. However, the frequency of use these implants show an upward trend, and the technology is developing rapidly. Nowadays, it is used more and more often during various traumatological surgeries of children [1].

Absorbable polymers have been used as surgical implants for more than three decades.

IntechOpen

In the case of first-generation polymers such as polyglycolic acid (PGA) and polylactic acid (PLA), several disadvantageous properties were experienced, such as too long absorption time and the appearance of adverse tissue reactions after implantation.

In the case of second-generation polymers, such as poly-L-lactide-co-glycolic acid (PLGA), such disadvantages do not have to be reckoned with. Among the biodegradable implants, pins, nails, various screws, and intramedullary nails are most often used.

PLGA does not cause adverse tissue reactions, but it slowly degrades as it reacts with the water in the human body. The large copolymer breaks down into its elements until, being an organic substance, carbon dioxide and water are produced, which leave the body physiologically. When developing absorbable implants, the basic goal was that the material to be implanted should have a high mechanical load capacity, but at the same time, during the physiological processes of bone healing, it would break down into its elements and be absorbed in the way described above. In the case of PLGA, an absorption time of 9–12 months was observed. Research on the absorption of PLGA implants has shown that the location of the canal is still visible on X-rays 2 years after implantation, but it disappears completely 3–4 years later. In some patients who underwent MRI several years after surgery, the results confirmed complete resorption of the implants. Further studies also confirmed that 2 years after the osteotomy of the pelvis, the canal left at the screw site was filled with bone tissue to 90%, and no tissue reactions were experienced during the degradation process [1–4].

The biggest advantage is that the removal of the implant is not necessary, thereby avoiding the possible complications associated with a second operation, including the risks that occur during anesthesia and surgery. In addition, we save children and parents from another hospital stay and mental burden.

Another potential benefit is slowing down the formation of bone bridges in the growth zone. The growth zone can be damaged not only by the fracture but also by the implant itself. In theory, absorbable implants can act as temporary space fillers in the growth zone while they degrade, thus slowing the formation of bone bridges and reducing the risk of growth disorders [2].

One of the major disadvantages of absorbable implants is that implants are currently extremely expensive. The costs are somewhat mitigated by the fact that a second operation is not necessary, which would also entail additional expenses.

Furthermore, it can be mentioned as a disadvantage that their load capacity and mechanical properties do not reach the level of metal implants.

One of the biggest difficulties in using PLGA implants is that most implants do not provide an X-ray shadow, so the surgeon performing the operation needs outstanding professional preparation and experience during the intervention.

Of all the implants, screws are the easiest to use. The reason for this is that they are cannulated, so the risk of possible complications can be reduced by using the guide wire. It is extremely important to prepare the screw with the correct size drill and tap, as these do not have a beam shadow, so accurate measurement and selection of the correct size screw are of utmost importance. The guide wire guides both the cannulated instruments and the screw.

Preparation is required to enter the PIN. Pre-drilling is performed with staple wires, and an absorbable implant of the appropriate size and thickness is introduced in their place.

Newer intramedullary implants can be used to treat fractures of the forearm and the wrist. The tip of the implant has a tricalcium phosphate marking that gives an X-ray shadow, which allows checking the position of the implant with the help of an image intensifier. During surgery, after the repair of the fracture, the medullary cavity must be prepared for the resorbable implant with special steel expansion devices. It is important to avoid high-energy movements when inserting the implant [5, 6].

The newly developed magnesium-based absorbable implants no longer require preparation, and due to their magnesium content, they also provide an X-ray shadow, so their position can be checked more easily under the X-ray [2, 7].

2. Clinical application of resorbable implants

2.1 Clavicle fracture

Conservative treatment is the most often chosen procedure for childhood clavicle fractures, however, in some cases, surgical intervention ensures a faster and more effective recovery. Relative indication of the operative method is more than 2 cm shortening and active sports activity.

Among surgical solutions, minimally invasive techniques such as elastic stable intramedullary nailing (ESIN), which is considered the gold-standard method, are preferred. Off label method uses resorbable intramedullary nail in some selected cases (**Figure 1**) [8].

Tips: Reposition often requires open reduction, and the insertion point of the absorbable implant is exactly the same as the elastic nailing.

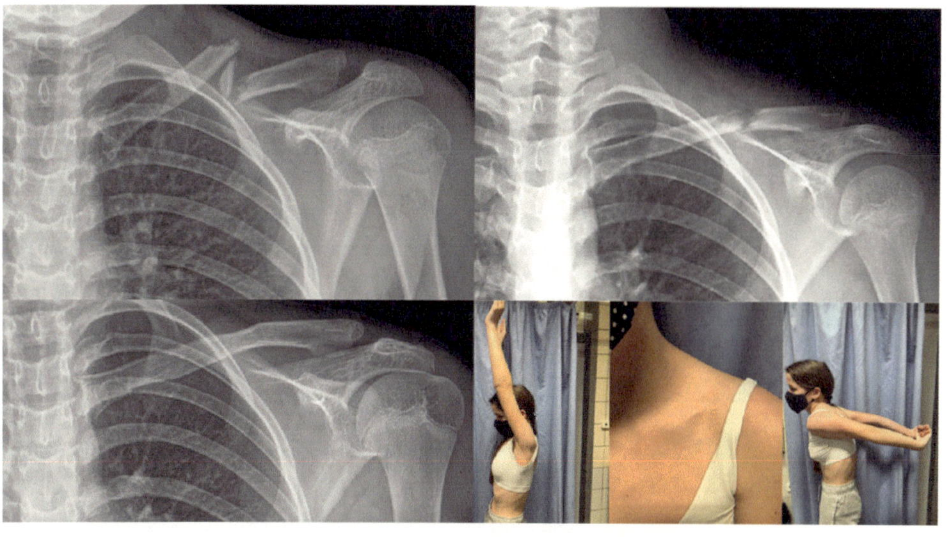

Figure 1.
A 9-year-old girl with left clavicle fracture, after open reduction and internal fixation by resorbable IM nail. One year later, the fracture is completely healed, and functional and cosmetic result was perfect.

2.2 Distal humeral fractures

Radial condyle fractures are the second most common type of injury among elbow fractures. It typically occurs in children between the ages of 2 and 10. Early diagnosis and, if necessary, surgical fixation and reconstruction of joint congruence are extremely important, thus reducing the risk of possible late complications. A growth disorder can occur as a serious complication, as a radial condyle fracture in childhood is characterized by the fact that it passes through the growth zone and affects the joint surface. In addition, pseudo-joints and bone death may also occur. Conservative therapy should be chosen in case of injuries with a displacement of less than 2 mm; however, another X-ray is recommended 5 days later. Several surgical techniques are available with the common goal of restoring joint congruence and avoiding late complications. In the case of fractures with minor displacement, percutaneous treatment is also a suitable alternative, however, many specialists prefer open reposition and internal fixation. Metal screws, K-wires, and resorbable screws and pins are the most common choices for fracture stabilization (**Figures 2** and **3**) [9–14].

Tips: After open exploration, we ensure the appropriate congruence of the articular surface. The achieved result is stabilized with temporary K-wires and then replaced with absorbable pins of the appropriate size. Stability is increased with a PDS loop.

Medial epicondyle fracture occurs when the forearm flexor muscles and the medial collateral ligament tear off the medial, ulnar apophysis of the humerus. The flexor muscle and the medial collateral ligament system of the elbow arise from this bone nucleus. This is the third most common elbow fracture, which occurs primarily in athletic adolescent boys (ages 9–14) in 75% of cases. The fracture is often, in half of the cases, accompanied by an elbow luxation. This type of fracture occurs because of valgus force when falling on an outstretched arm. Surgery is warranted if the fracture

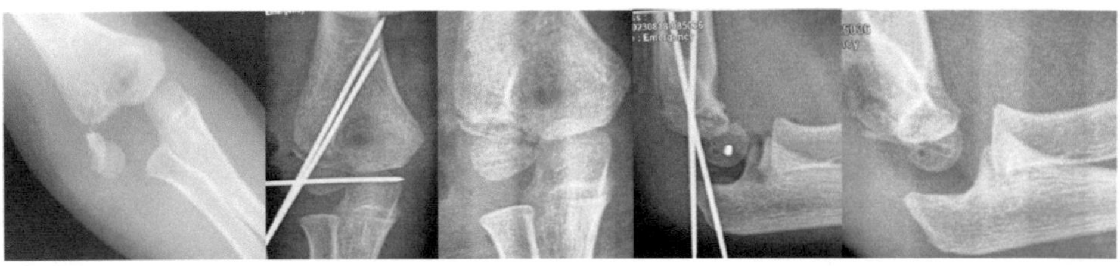

Figure 2.
Displaced lateral humeral condyle fracture of the humerus. Open reduction and transient fixation by K-wires and the same view of X-rays with the fracture fixed by resorbable pins and PDS loop.

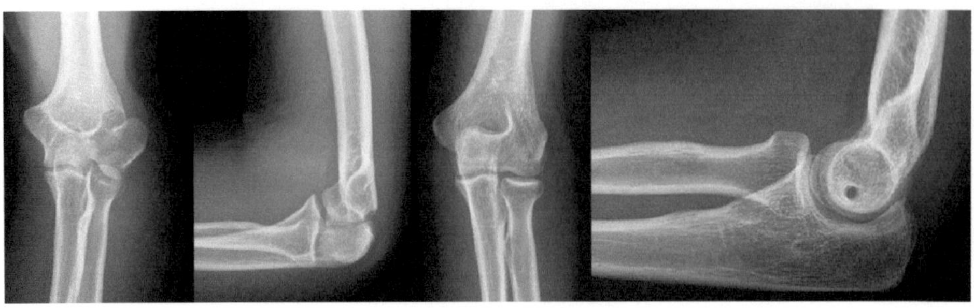

Figure 3.
Dislocated lateral humeral condyle fracture treated by two resorbable screws.

is open or if the broken piece of bone is wedged into the joint. In addition, surgery is an absolute indication if the fracture is accompanied by an elbow luxation, if the ulnar nerve is affected (numbness, tingling), or if, based on imaging, the displacement exceeds 15 mm, or there is instability of the elbow joint. If the radiograph shows a nondisplaced fracture, conservative therapy is the recommended treatment. However, the optimal treatment approach for fractures with minor displacement remains controversial. The operation is performed with an open reduction, where the protection of the ulnar nerve and the precise reduction and stable fixation of the medial epicondyle are of utmost importance. The reconstruction can be performed in different ways, with metal implants (K-wire, screw) or absorbable implants (pin, screw) (**Figure 4**). The surgical technique does not necessarily affect the result, and in the case of metal implants, a second operation is necessary to remove them [15–18].

Tips: After isolating the ulnar nerve, the fragment is precisely re-inserted in its original place, its size determines the type of absorbable implant. A screw is recommended for a larger fragment, while a pin is recommended for a smaller fragment.

Capitellum fractures in pediatric patients are uncommon and difficult to diagnose, with treatment outcomes varying based on the promptness of diagnosis and the chosen treatment approach. Additionally, there is a limited body of research on the management of capitellum fractures, with most studies consisting of case reports or small case series. The treatment of displaced anterior and posterolateral shear injuries (type-Ib and type-IIb, respectively) typically involves surgical fixation. Several techniques have been reported, including suture repair, Kirschner wire fixation, bioabsorbable pin fixation (**Figure 5**), and the use of cortical, cannulated, or variable-pitch headless compression screws. To date, no studies have directly compared the outcomes of these different fixation methods. As a result, the choice of

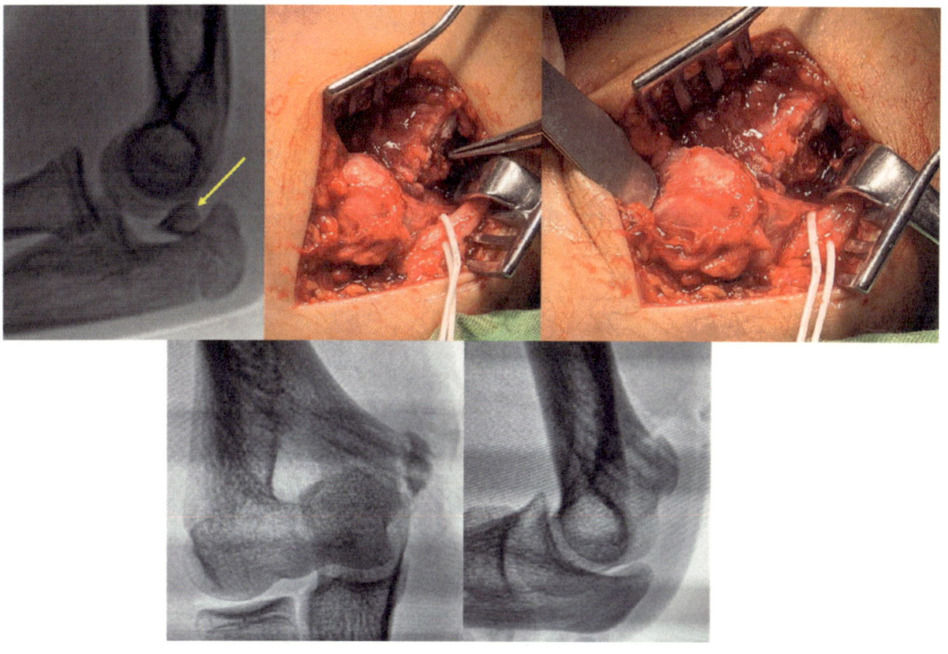

Figure 4.
The yellow arrow shows the medial epicondyle dislocated into the joint. Intraoperative pictures present the fracture side and the fragment. Postoperative X-rays show the fracture stabilized with resorbable implants (screw) in a good position.

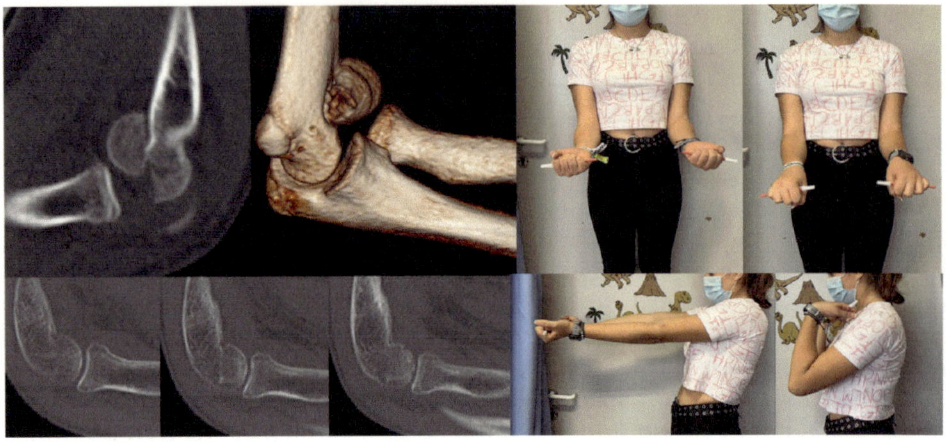

Figure 5.
Displaced capitellum fracture preop CT and 1 year later control CT showed perfect articular surface and healed fracture. The fracture was fixed by open reduction and resorbable pin fixation. The patient healed with full function.

fixation technique is largely at the surgeon's discretion, based on their experience and the specific characteristics of the fracture [19].

Tips: In the case of exploration, the implants guided from the anterior surface can be sunk under the cartilage, so they do not cause any irritation on the opposing articular surface.

2.3 Fractures around elbow joint

Radial head and neck fractures account for up to 14% of all pediatric elbow fractures and pose a significant challenge in treating young patients. In as many as 39% of proximal radius fractures, there may be an associated fracture that can easily be missed on initial standard radiographs. Treatment options for proximal radius fractures in children vary, ranging from non-surgical approaches like immobilization alone or closed reduction followed by immobilization, to more invasive procedures such as closed reduction with percutaneous pinning or open reduction with internal fixation (K-wires, resorbable pins (**Figure 6**), and mini screws) [20, 21].

Tips: Reconstruction of the joint surface is the most important. The implants can be sunk under the cartilage and compression can be created by using the nails.

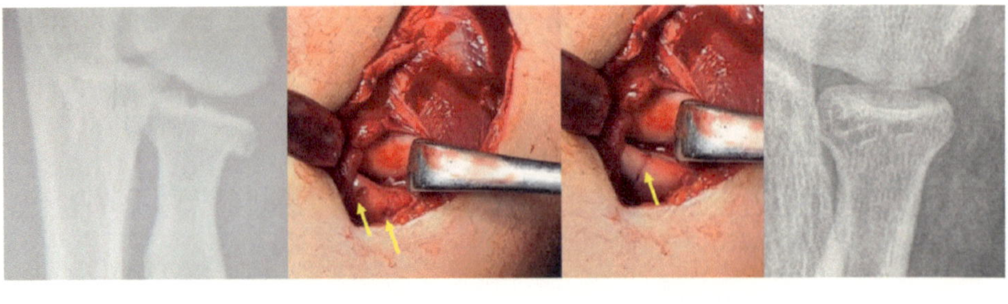

Figure 6.
Radial head intraarticular fracture preop ap X-ray, intraoperative pictures show two pins (yellow narrow) and good reduction (yellow narrow), and correct articular congruency. Postop X-ray shows good position of the radial head, congruent articular surface.

2.4 Olecranon

Olecranon fractures make up 4% of all pediatric elbow fractures and are associated with other ipsilateral elbow injuries in up to 20% of cases. These associated injuries are often linked to worse outcomes. In pediatric patients, surgical indications are less well-defined, and there is often uncertainty about the best surgical technique to use in a growing skeleton with an open physis. The long-term effects of olecranon fractures involving the physis, as well as the potential complications of surgical hardware such as wires crossing the physis, remain unclear [22, 23]. There is no evidence of how you do can treat these patient, one option is to use resorbable pins and PDS compression loop (**Figure 7**).

Tips: The step of the operation is the same as the K-wire and cerclage technique, and there is no difference in the postoperative period. Very good indication that there is no differences of metal procedure.

2.5 Forearm fractures

Among long bone fractures, childhood forearm fractures are the most common and account for approximately half of all childhood fractures. About 20% of forearm fractures affect the body of the bone, i.e., the diaphysis. The incidence of fractures increases for both sexes until the age of 11–12 and then decreases for girls, while it continues to rise for boys. These injuries are often caused by a direct or indirect mechanism, because of a fall on the hand or forearm. The most common causes include sports and recreational activities such as cycling, rollerblading, and ball sports, where children often fall by extending their arms for protection. This injury mechanism is known as "fall on outstretched hand" (FOOSH).

In case of fractures with significant dislocation, instability, open injuries, or severe soft tissue damage, operative treatment is warranted. In children, a minimally invasive method, the elastic titanium medullary nailing, comes to the fore, which differs from the treatment of adults. Implantation and removal of the titanium elastic nail is less invasive than plate fixation. One of the biggest advantages of this metal implant is that there is no need for external fixation after surgery, as it provides a high degree of stability, making the postoperative period much more child friendly. The indication for the use of absorbable implants has expanded in recent years, so childhood forearm fractures are increasingly treated with absorbable implants (**Figure 8**). Unlike children treated with metal implants, external fixation is also required, the form and time of which is not yet clear. In 2020, an international scientific working group was formed to assess the treatment of childhood forearm fractures with absorbable implants. The advantage of the method is that it does not require metal removal or

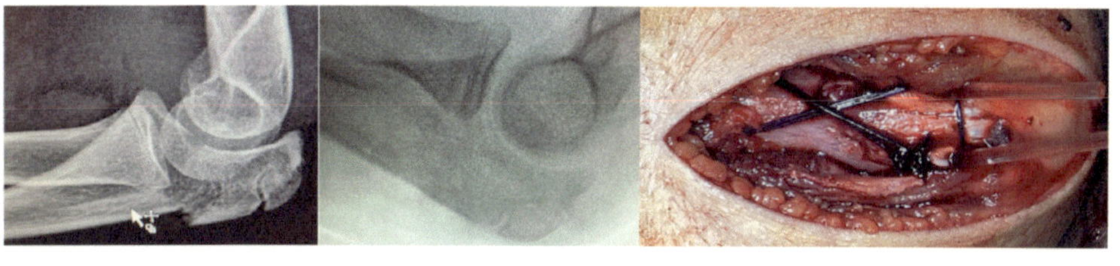

Figure 7.
Olecranon fracture primary lateral X-ray. Postop X-ray shows perfect articular surface, and intraoperative picture shows two resorbable pins and PDS loop fixation.

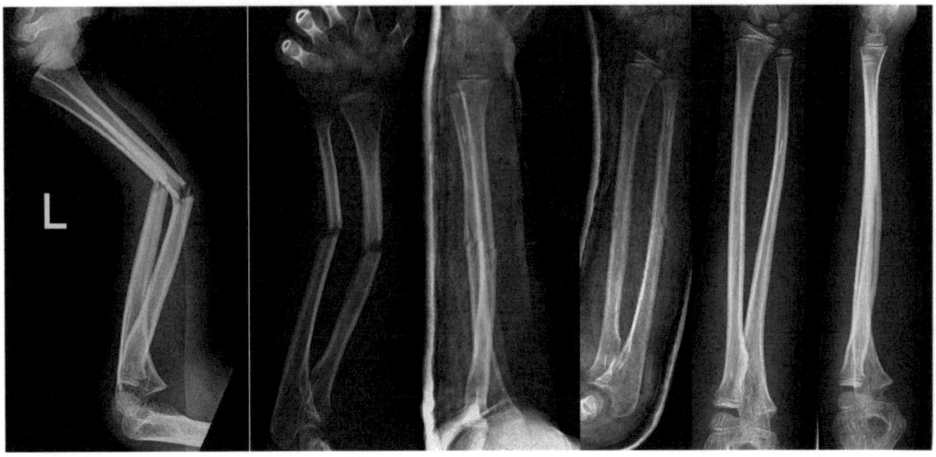

Figure 8.
Left diaphyseal forearm fracture, after reduction and resorbable IM nail fixation. Two years later, the X-ray shows completely healed fracture with no sign of growth disturbance or residual deformity.

re-anesthesia. The disadvantage in the case of forearm fractures is that additional plaster fixation is required [5, 24–27].

Tips: The medullary cavity must be prepared to receive the resorbable implant, which may present more difficulties. The narrow medullary cavity often causes technical difficulties. In the case of fractures that are difficult to reduce, the introduction of an absorbable implant is not easy. The stabilization of the fracture is not as great as in the case of the elastic nail, which is why additional plaster fixation is necessary. The course of surgery and the insertion points of the implants are the same as traditional elastic nailing.

2.6 Distal radial fracture

Among the fractures that occur frequently in children is the distal radius fracture, which is one of the most common types of fractures in children. However, there is still no uniform professional consensus regarding its treatment. If the fracture involves significant displacement or shortening, it must be treated operatively. The most common method of fracture fixation is closed reduction and percutaneous fixation with a Kirschner wire, which is a simple and cost-effective procedure, this method has many potential complications (skin irritation, K-wire migration, and superficial wound infection), but there are also alternative solutions [28, 29]. For dia- and metaphysis fractures, it is possible to stabilize with elastic nails, but more recently, the short absorbable IM-Nail has also become a suitable option (**Figure 9**) [6].

Tips: In the case of completely dislocated fractures, after reposition, intramedullary fixation bent in a short c-shape is an easily performed surgical technique with good results with sufficient practice. It provides good stability, and fewer complications should be expected than with K-wire fixation.

2.7 Fractures around knee joint

Patella fractures in children can be classified into three main types: fractures of the corpus of the patella, i.e., the body of the bone, pole dislocation, and osteochondral fractures. These fracture types differ not only in the mechanism of injury, but also in

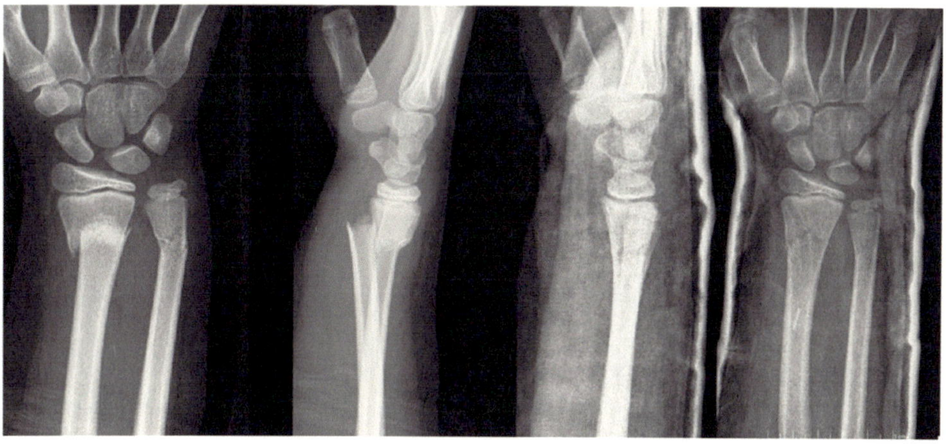

Figure 9.
Distal forearm fracture. Fully displaced (overriding) metaphyseal radius fracture associated with stable greenstick ulna metaphyseal fracture. After reduction and short intramedullary resorbable nailing fixation of the radius.

treatment options. In osteochondral fractures, the detached cartilage surface, which contains both bone and spongiosa, is visible, although only the bony part is visible on X-rays. In the case of this type of fracture, surgical intervention is essential, as the presence of a free articular fragment can lead to serious consequences without treatment.

In the case of a larger fragment, it is possible to reattach it using metal or absorbable implants (**Figure 10**).

In the case of patella dislocation, the rate of occurrence of osteochondral fractures is 70%. As the patella shifts laterally, shear forces act on the medial surface of the patella and the lateral surface of the femoral condyle (**Figure 11**). In almost half of the patella luxation occurring in childhood, the root cause is a sports accident during some physical activity or playing ball. In 95% of cases, the injury also affects the

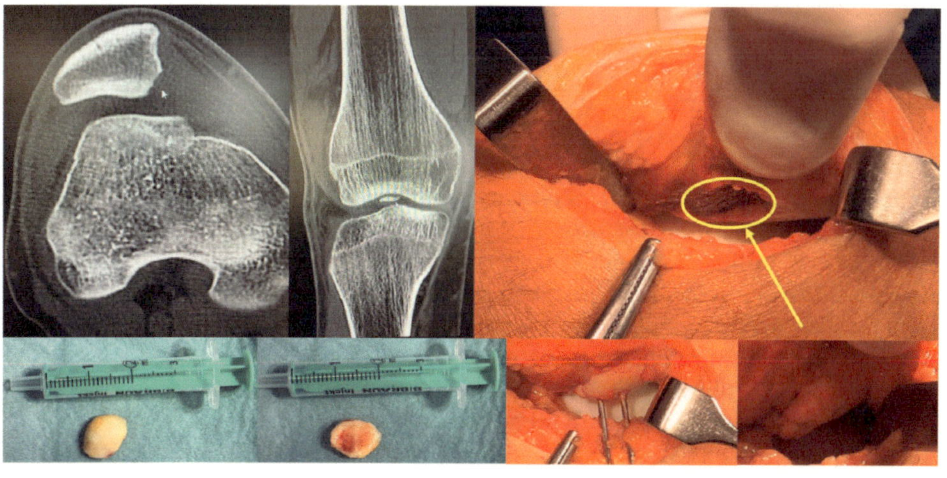

Figure 10.
Patella osteochondral fracture after patella dislocation. Intraoperative pictures show the defect and the size of the osteochondral fragment. Temporary fixation with K-wires and finally resorbable implants fix the fragment in a correct position.

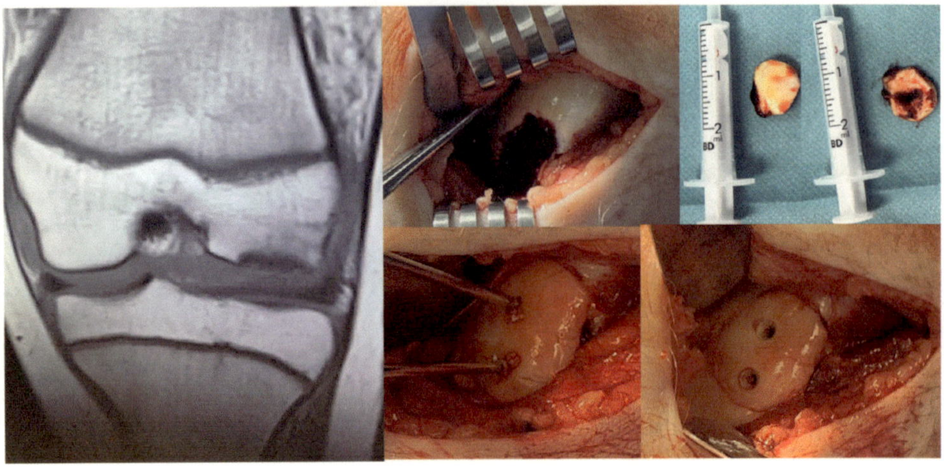

Figure 11.
Femur lateral osteochondral fracture preoperative MR picture, intraoperative pictures show the defect and size of the fragment. Transient fixation by K-wire and final fixation by resorbable nails.

medial patellofemoral ligament. In almost every case, we can encounter some anatomical predisposition that predisposes to the development of the injury [30–35].

Tips: Regardless of the size of the osteochondral fragment, resorbable implants are an excellent solution for fixing the fracture after the fractured fragment has been repaired.

2.8 Tibial tubercle fractures

Injuries of the tuberositas tibiae are rare in children, accounting for less than 1% of all physical injuries; however, their frequency increases with age due to participation in various sports activities. It is most common among adolescents aged 12–16, as the apophysis is most vulnerable at that time. Boys are primarily affected; this can be explained by the fact that the proximal physis closes later and they participate more often in sports activities.

This type of fracture occurs when the quadriceps contract forcefully against resistance, such as during a jump, or when there is a rapid knee bend during landing with a contracted quadriceps. Therefore, sports involving jumping, such as basketball, high jump, sprinting, football, increase the risk of this injury. Fractures accompanied by displacement, as well as fractures involving the secondary bone core and joint of the proximal epiphysis (Ogden III A, B, IV, V injuries) are an absolute indication for surgery, the aim of which is precise anatomical reposition. Metal implants are primarily used for operative fracture treatment, which provide adequate stability for primary bone healing. Nowadays we use absorbable screws more and more often (**Figure 12**) [2, 36].

Tips: Surgical exploration and the technique are the same when using a metal implant. The same stability as with metal implants can be achieved.

2.9 Ankle fractures

Ankle fractures account for approximately 5% of all childhood fractures. 15–20% of growth cartilage injuries affect the distal end of the tibia, making it the third most

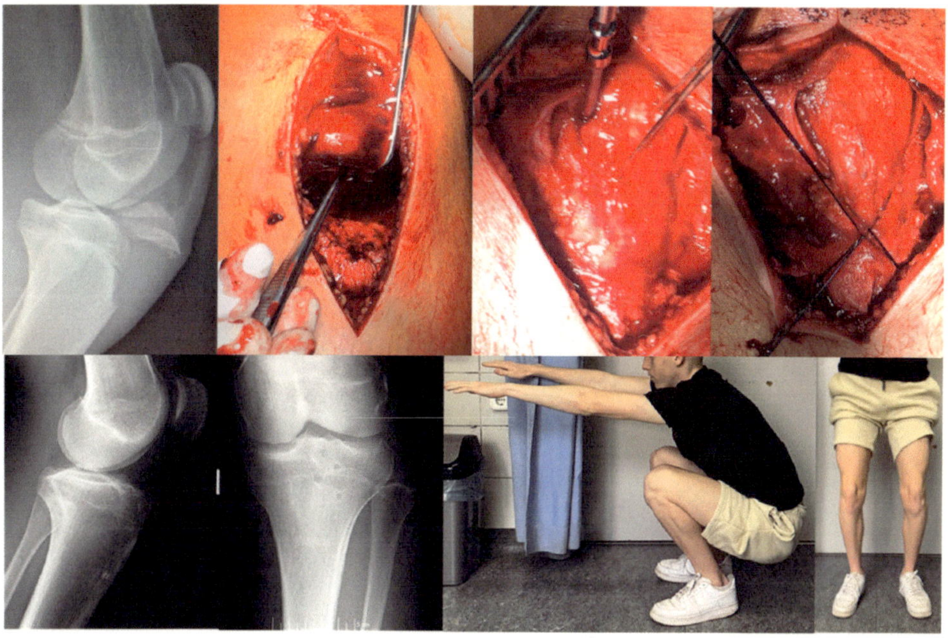

Figure 12.
Abruption of tibial tubercle, open reduction, and internal fixation by resorbable screws and PDS loop. One year after the operation, the patient returned to the sport. The fracture is healed physically and radiologically too.

common after phalanx and distal radius fractures. Ankle injuries are most common in children between the ages of 8 and 15. It is twice as common in boys, which can partly be explained by the later closure of the physis. It follows from the peculiarities of the immature skeletal system in childhood that even a low-energy trauma to the ankle can lead to a fracture, because the ankle ligaments connected to the epiphysis of the tibia and tibia are much stronger than the open physis. It follows that the growth cartilage is more exposed to the effects of shearing forces and rotational mechanisms, so that most of the time the bone is damaged, while the ligaments remain intact. In adolescence, with the beginning of ossification of the growth zone, characteristic fracture types may develop. In the 18-month period before the complete closure of the distal physis of the tibia, the medial part of the physis has already ossified, but the lateral part remains open. During this period, the so-called transitional fractures include triplane and juvenile Tillaux fractures (**Figure 13**). A triplane fracture occurs early in the fusion of the physis, usually because of a supination-rotation mechanism. It is a complex, three-plane SH-IV fracture. The physis breaks in a transverse plane, the coronal plane touches the metaphysis of the tibia, and the sagittal plane extends through the epiphysis to the palatal surface. Surgical treatment of Salter-Harris type I and II injuries is only necessary if they are associated with large displacement or significant axis deviation. Even after the repair, the stability is not adequate, or fractures that cannot be repaired under cover also require surgery. The surgical indication for Salter-Harris III and IV fractures is in the case of joint step formation exceeding 2 millimeters and/or joint space greater than 2 millimeters. Open fractures in the second or third degree, as well as fractures with vascular or nerve damage, regardless of their type, constitute an absolute indication for surgery. In the surgical treatment of ankle fractures, metal screw osteosynthesis is widely known and the first procedure of choice. When resorbable implants were developed, the primary goal was to

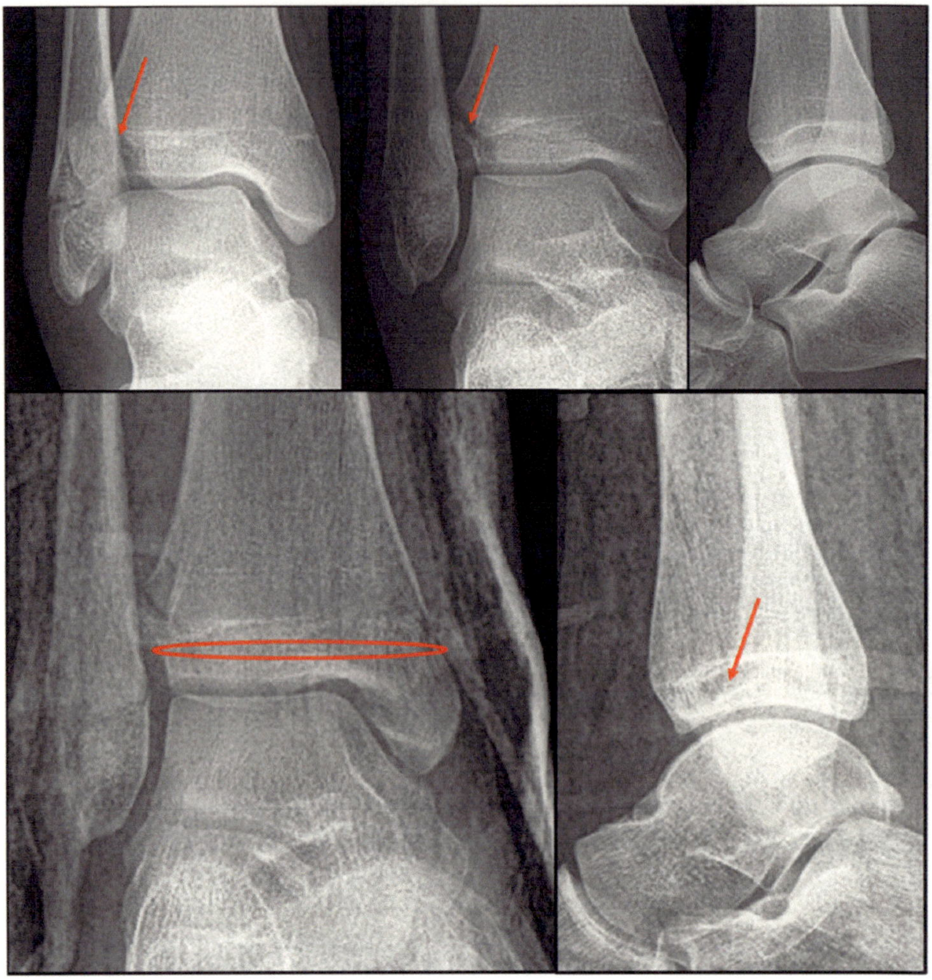

Figure 13.
Distal tibial fracture (Tillaux fracture: red narrow shows the fracture gap). Postoperative X-rays show good articular congruency. Red ellipsis shows the resorbable screw position (shadow screw).

avoid the need for another surgical intervention to remove the devices. The implants are made of a special biodegradable polymer that is designed to maintain its stability until the fracture heals and then be absorbed by the body. Thanks to this, during the degradation of the screw, the load is gradually transferred to the bone tissue, thereby promoting remodeling, eliminating the negative consequences experienced with metal screws [2, 37, 38].

Tips: The most accepted and most widespread indication area.

Screws can be inserted using a percutaneous technique. The most important step is the exact reposition of the fracture, which is held by the absorbable screw.

3. Conclusions

With absorbable implants, more and more childhood fractures can be treated with good results. The authors described the most common pediatric fracture types, in which the same good results can be achieved with an absorbable implant as with metal, titanium implants, which are currently considered the gold standard. Based on the clinical results so far (short- and medium-term follow-up of the patients), it can be said that the new methods enabled similarly stable fixation as the fixation with metal implants, which is considered the gold standard. A distinct advantage over these procedures is that there is no need to remove the implant, thus avoiding a second operation and reducing the risk of surgical complications. It is also a positive thing that absorbable implants can be sunk into the marrow cavity of the bone, they can easily be dropped under the skin, so they do not cause soft tissue irritation. The healthcare system is also not burdened with the costs of the second surgery (metal removal) and the associated hospital care. The only drawback of the method is the price of the implants.

Conflict of interest

The authors declare no conflict of interest.

Author details

Gergo Jozsa[1*] and Marcell Varga[2]

1 Division of Surgery, Traumatology and Otorhinolaryngology, Department of Paediatrics, Clinical Complex, University of Pécs, Pécs, Hungary

2 Department of Pediatric Traumatology, Péterfy Hospital, Manninger Jenő National Trauma Center, Budapest, Hungary

*Address all correspondence to: jozsa.gergo@pte.hu

IntechOpen

© 2025 The Author(s). Licensee IntechOpen. This chapter is distributed under the terms of the Creative Commons Attribution License (http://creativecommons.org/licenses/by/4.0), which permits unrestricted use, distribution, and reproduction in any medium, provided the original work is properly cited.

References

[1] Rocha CV, Gonçalves V, da Silva MC, Bañobre-López M, Gallo J. PLGA-based composites for various biomedical applications. International Journal of Molecular Sciences. 2022;**23**(4):2034. DOI: 10.3390/ijms23042034

[2] Heye P, Matissek C, Seidl C, Varga M, Kassai T, Jozsa G, et al. Making hardware removal unnecessary by using resorbable implants for osteosynthesis in children. Children. 2022;**9**:471. DOI: 10.3390/children9040471

[3] Grün NG, Holweg PL, Donohue N, Klestil T, Weinberg AM. Resorbable implants in pediatric fracture treatment. Innovative Surgical Sciences. 2018;**3**(2):119-125

[4] Rokkanen PU, Böstman O, Hirvensalo E, Mäkelä EA, Partio EK, Pätiälä H, et al. Bioabsorbable fixation in orthopaedic surgery and traumatology. Biomaterials. 2000;**21**(24):2607-2613

[5] Dávid ÁL, Mucsina F, Antal E, Lamberti AG, Lőrincz A, Józsa G. Comparison of titanium versus resorbable intramedullary nailing in pediatric forearm fractures. Children (Basel). 2024;**11**(8):942. DOI: 10.3390/children11080942

[6] Varga M, Józsa G, Hanna D, Tóth M, Hajnal B, Krupa Z, et al. Bioresorbable implants vs. Kirschner-wires in the treatment of severely displaced distal paediatric radius and forearm fractures—A retrospective multicentre study. BMC Musculoskeletal Disorders. 2022;**23**:362

[7] Tsakiris V, Tardei C, Clicinschi FM. Biodegradable Mg alloys for orthopedic implants—A review. Journal of Magnesium and Alloys. 2021;**9**(6):1884-1905. DOI: 10.1016/j.jma.2021.06.024

[8] Markes AR, Garcia-Lopez E, Halvorson RT, Swarup I. Management of displaced Midshaft clavicle fractures in pediatrics and adolescents: Operative vs nonoperative treatment. Orthopedic Research and Reviews. 2022;**14**:373-381. DOI: 10.2147/ORR.S340538

[9] Ganeshalingam R, Donnan A, Evans O, Hoq M, Camp M, Donnan L. Lateral condylar fractures of the humerus in children: Does the type of fixation matter? The Bone & Joint Journal. 2018;**100-B**(3):387-395. DOI: 10.1302/0301-620X.100B3.BJJ-2017-0814.R1

[10] Schlitz RS, Schwertz JM, Eberhardt AW, Gilbert SR. Biomechanical analysis of screws versus K-wires for lateral humeral condyle fractures. Journal of Pediatric Orthopedics. 2015;**35**(8):e93-e97. DOI: 10.1097/BPO.0000000000000450

[11] Rehm A, Thahir A, Granger L, Ashby E. Impacts of fracture types on success rate of closed reduction and percutaneous pinning in pediatric lateral condyle humerus fractures displaced >4 mm. Journal of Pediatric Orthopaedics. 2023;**43**(2):e190-e191. DOI: 10.1097/BPO.0000000000002233

[12] Raghavan R, Jones A, Dwyer AJ. Should Kirschner wires for fixation of lateral humeral condyle fractures in children be buried or left exposed? A systematic review. Orthopaedics & Traumatology, Surgery & Research. 2019;**105**(4):739-745. DOI: 10.1016/j.otsr.2019.03.007. Epub 2019

[13] Cummings JL, Schwabe MT, Rivera AE, Sanders J, Denning JR,

Neal K, et al. K-wire versus screw fixation in displaced lateral condyle fractures of the humerus in children: A multicenter study of 762 fractures. Journal of Pediatric Orthopaedics. 1 Apr 2023;**43**(4):e284-e289. DOI: 10.1097/BPO.0000000000002348. Epub 2023 Jan 11. PMID: 36634213; PMCID: PMC11216759

[14] Kassai T, Krupa Z, Józsa G, Hanna D, Varga M. Comparison of biodegradable and metallic tension-band fixation for paediatric lateral condyle fracture of the elbow. Injury. 2024;**55 Suppl 3**:111403. DOI: 10.1016/j.injury.2024.111403. Epub 2024 Sep 17

[15] Kassai T, Varga M, Józsa G. Pediatric medial humeral epicondyle fracture in children: Are biodegradable pins with tension band absorbable sutures efficient? Medicine (Baltimore). 2022;**101**(30):e29817. DOI: 10.1097/MD.0000000000029817

[16] Su Y, Nan G. Treatment of medial humeral epicondyle fractures in children using absorbable self-reinforced polylactide pins. Medicine (Baltimore). 2020;**99**(17):19861

[17] Hughes M, Dua K, O'Hara NN, Brighton BK, et al. Variation among pediatric orthopaedic surgeons when treating medial epicondyle fractures. Journal of Pediatric Orthopedics. 2019;**39**:592-596

[18] Firth AM, Marson BA, Hunter JB. Paediatric medial humeral epicondyle fracture management: 2019 approach. Current Opinion in Pediatrics. 2019;**31**:86-91

[19] Yang D, Baghdadi S, Värk P-R, Buttrick E, Shah AS. Classification and treatment of pediatric capitellar fractures. Journal of Pediatric Orthopaedics. 2024;**44**(6):358-365. DOI: 10.1097/BPO.0000000000002650

[20] Macken AA, Eygendaal D, van Bergen CJ. Diagnosis, treatment and complications of radial head and neck fractures in the pediatric patient. World Journal of Orthopedics. 2022;**13**:238-249. DOI: 10.5312/wjo.v13.i3.238

[21] Ackerson R, Nguyen A, Carry PM, Pritchard B, Hadley-Miller N, Scott F. Intra-articular radial head fractures in the skeletally immature patient: Complications and management. Journal of Pediatric Orthopedics. 2015;**35**:443. DOI: 10.1097/BPO.0000000000000302

[22] Holme TJ, Karbowiak M, Arnander M, Gelfer Y. Paediatric olecranon fractures: A systematic review. EFORT Open Reviews. 2020;**5**(5):280-288. DOI: 10.1302/2058-5241.5.190082

[23] Scheider P, Ganger R, Farr S. Complications of hardware removal in pediatric upper limb surgery: A retrospective single-center study of 317 patients. Medicine. 2020;**99**(5):e19010. DOI: 10.1097/MD.0000000000019010

[24] Korhonen L, Perhomaa M, Kyrö A, Pokka T, Serlo W, Merikanto J, et al. Intramedullary nailing of forearm shaft fractures by biodegradable compared with titanium nails: Results of a prospective randomized trial in children with at least two years of follow-up. Biomaterials. 2018;**185**:383-392

[25] Lascombes P, Prevot J, Ligier JN, Metaizeau JP, Poncelet T. Elastic stable intramedullary nailing in forearm shaft fractures in children: 85 cases. Journal of Pediatric Orthopedics. 1990;**10**:167-171

[26] Perhomaa M, Pokka T, Korhonen L, Kyrö A, Niinimäki J, Serlo W, et al. Randomized controlled trial of the clinical recovery and biodegradation of polylactide-co-glycolide implants used in the intramedullary nailing of children's forearm shaft fractures with at least four

years of follow-up. Journal of Clinical Medicine. 2021;**10**:995

[27] Sinikumpu JJ, Keränen J, Haltia AM, Serlo W, Merikanto J. A new mini-invasive technique in treating pediatric diaphyseal forearm fractures by bioabsorbable elastic stable intramedullary nailing: A preliminary technical report. Scandinavian Journal of Surgery. 2013;**102**:258-264

[28] Khandekar S, Tolessa E, Jones S. Displaced distal end radius fractures in children treated with Kirschner wires—A systematic review. Acta Orthopaedica Belgica. 2016;**82**(4):681-689

[29] Dua K, Stein MK, O'Hara NN, Brighton BK, Hennrikus WL, Herman MJ, et al. Variation among pediatric orthopaedic surgeons when diagnosing and treating pediatric and adolescent distal radius fractures. Journal of Pediatric Orthopedics. 2019;**39**(6):306-313. DOI: 10.1097/BPO.0000000000000954

[30] Sinikumpu JJ, Serlo W. Biodegradable poly-L-lactide-co-glycolide copolymer pin fixation of a traumatic patellar osteochondral fragment in an 11-year-old child: A novel surgical approach. Experimental and Therapeutic Medicine. 2017;**13**:242-246

[31] Gkiokas A, Morassi LG, Kohl S, Zampakides C, Megremis P, Evangelopoulos DS. Bioabsorbable pins for treatment of osteochondral fractures of the knee after acute patella dislocation in children and young adolescents. Advances in Orthopedics. 2012;**2012**:e249687. DOI: 10.1155/2012/249687

[32] Sari E. Delayed osteochondral fracture fixation of the knee in a pediatric patient. Turkish Journal of Trauma and Emergency Surgery. 2020;**27**:369-373. DOI: 10.14744/tjtes.2020.59056

[33] Agrawal U, Tiwari V, Selvanayagam R. A rare case of large osteochondral fracture of patella. Cureus. 2023;**15**:e41245. DOI: 10.7759/cureus.41245

[34] Bauer KL. Osteochondral injuries of the knee in pediatric patients. The Journal of Knee Surgery. 2018;**31**:382-391. DOI: 10.1055/s-0038-1625956

[35] Kühle J, Angele P, Balcarek P, Eichinger M, Feucht M, Haasper C, et al. Treatment of osteochondral fractures of the knee: A meta-analysis of available scientific evidence. International Orthopaedics. 2013;**37**:2385-2394. DOI: 10.1007/s00264-013-2070-7

[36] Reyes CD, Wu W, Pandya NK. Adolescent tibial tubercle fracture: Review of outcomes and complications. Current Reviews in Musculoskeletal Medicine. 2023;**16**:392-397. DOI: 10.1007/s12178-023-09849-9

[37] Nudelman H, Lőrincz A, Lamberti AG, Varga M, Kassai T, Józsa G. Management of pediatric ankle fractures: Comparison of biodegradable PLGA implants with traditional metal screws. Frontiers in Pediatrics. 2024;**12**:1410750. DOI: 10.3389/fped.2024.1410750

[38] Podeszwa DA, Wilson PL, Holland AR, Copley LAB. Comparison of bioabsorbable versus metallic implant fixation for physeal and epiphyseal fractures of the distal tibia. Journal of Pediatric Orthopedics. 2008;**28**(8):859-863. DOI: 10.1097/BPO.0b013e31818e19d7

Chapter 4

Distal Biceps Tendon Repair: Surgical Techniques

Triantafyllos Katsimentzas, Athina-Zacharoula Ditsiou, Vasileios Balamotis and Konstantinos Ditsios

Abstract

Traumatic lesions of the distal biceps brachii are uncommon. They often result from rapid elbow flexion against resistance. Although several pathogenic theories have been proposed, the hypovascular zone hypothesis seems to be the most valid. Both conservative and surgical approaches have been proposed. Conservative treatment is only indicated in low-demanding patients and in those who have severe comorbidities. Regarding the surgical approach for acute ruptures, three options are available: the single-, the double-incision and the endoscopic techniques. In cases of chronic tears, it is typically necessary to utilize a graft to bridge the gap created by tendon retraction. In this chapter, we will describe the anatomy, pathophysiology, symptoms and imaging of this lesion, but especially the possible surgical techniques that exist in the international bibliography.

Keywords: distal biceps tear, single-incision, dual-incision, endoscopic, chronic distal biceps tear

1. Introduction

Rupture of the distal biceps tendon is a relatively rare incident and usually occurs after insignificant tension is applied to the tendon (Koch). It affects commonly the dominant extremity in male population around their fourth decade; women are sparsely reported, and the overall incidence is 1.2 per 100,000 population [1]. Risk factors associated with spontaneous tendon ruptures are smoking, obesity, corticosteroids and anabolic steroids, while less common factors include statins and quinolones, gout, diabetes and chronic kidney disease [2, 3].

1.1 Anatomy

The biceps brachii is one of the three main muscles that form the anterior compartment of the arm. It serves as a flexor of the arm and elbow, is the main supinator of the forearm and is innervated by the musculocutaneous nerve, originating from C5 to C7 cervical nerve roots [2]. The whole musculotendinous units involve two distinct, parallel parts: the long head of biceps, which arises from the superior lip of the glenoid coursing in the radial side of the arm and the short head arising from the coracoid process and remaining at the ulnar side. The distal biceps tendon is formed by the junction of the short and long heads of the muscle distally, and it follows a path through the antecubital fossa to insert on the ulnar side of radial tuberosity [4].

The bicipital aponeurosis, also known as the lacertus fibrosus, originates from the distal biceps tendon (DBT) at the level of the musculotendinous junction. It consists of three layers and spreads in a medial and distal direction to join the antebrachial fascia. It completely envelopes the forearm flexor muscles as well as the median nerve and brachial artery and attaches eventually to the radial and ulnar side of the ulna [5]. Conflicting reports exist regarding the origin of lacertus fibrosus in the cadaveric study of Eames; it is stated that the superficial and deep layer of the aponeurosis originates from the radial side of the long head of the biceps at the level of the muscolotendinous junction [5]. In contrast, the bicipital aponeurosis was studied and found to originate from the proximal aspect of the short head of the distal tendon in all specimens studied in the cadaveric study of Atwal. The authors also concluded that this might be useful in helping to identify the short-head distal tendon unit and proceed to an anatomical surgical repair [6].

The tendon's cross-section at the level beyond the aponeurosis is oval with an average width of 5.3 mm, and it flattens and broads to 19.2 mm as it courses more distally to its insertional point. The anteroposterior diameter was larger in the right elbows, an evident corresponding to the dominant hand; male cadavers also presented thicker and wider tendons, while there was no difference regarding the insertional site size between males and females [7].

The trajectory of the two muscle bellies of biceps brachii that form distinct parts of the distal biceps tendon on the radial tuberosity has become evident thanks to anatomical studies [5, 6]. The DBT rotates 90° externally from its origin to insertion [6, 7]. In two cadaveric studies, in 20 out of 32 specimens, both muscle bellies and their corresponding distal tendons demonstrated an individual course, and even in the other 12 specimens, their tendons could be grossly divided [5, 6]. After externally rotating, the anterior part of the distal biceps tendon, which derives from the short head, inserts more distally at the radial tuberosity and serves as a powerful flexor of the elbow, whereas the posterior part, which derives from the long head, inserts more proximally and further laterally from the rotation axis of radius in the radial tuberosity, serving predominately as a strong supinator of the antebrachium [5].

In the cadaveric study of Mazzocca et al., the anatomy of bicipital tuberosity is thoroughly described. The mean length of the bicpes tendon (BT) is 22 mm, mean width 15 mm and the BT ridge, which is of great importance, is absent in 6%, bifid in 6% and characterized as small, medium or large in 88%. The torsional anatomy of BT is also defined by a line parallel to the long axis of the tuberosity and a line that bisects the radial styloid so that the BT-radial styloid angle is found to be on average 123° (**Figure 1**) [4].

The footprint of the tendon at the posterior rim of the radial tuberosity is described as long, thin, vertical, and semilunar, with no intraosseous prolongation of fibers [7]. The most proximal point of the insertion site from the radial head articular margin is on average 23 mm, length and width of the footprint average 21 and 7 mm, respectively, covering an area of approximately 108mm^2 (60mm^2 for the short head and 48mm^2 for the long head) [6]. Unmatched findings are reported in the

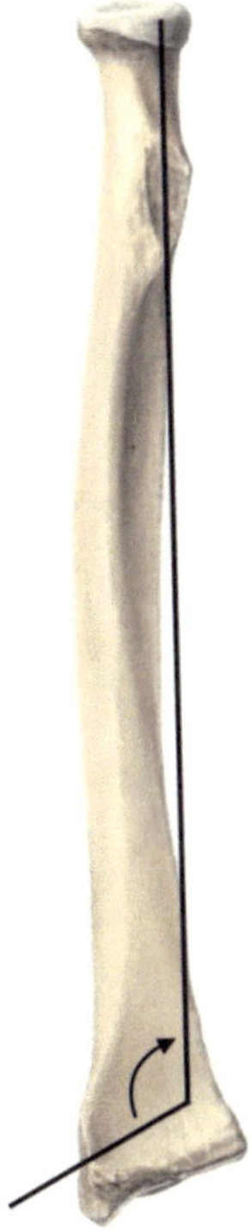

Figure 1.
Bone anatomy.

study of Eames, the study of Mazzocca and the one of Koch regarding the footprint size of each distal tendon [4, 5]. Eames et al. described an oval-shaped insertional site of the long-head distal tendon, which occupies most of the radial tuberosity, and a smaller fan-like insertional site of the short-head distal tendon [5]. Mazzocca et al., in their cadaveric study, found an average DBT length and width of 14 and 32 mm, respectively, with the insertion occupying 63% and 13% of the tuberosity's length and width, respectively [4]. Finally, Koch et al. report on a footprint size of 3cm^2 (**Figure 2**) [8].

A bicipital bursa, a thin layer of synovial membrane-like tissue, is always present surrounding the insertional site and is attached proximally to the radial side of the DBT and fans distally on the ulnar side encircling completely the DBT [5, 8]. It can be found in the raphe between the DBT and brachialis muscle when the elbow is extended and between the DBT and radial bone when pronation is applied [5].

The vascular anatomy relevant to the biceps insertion site is significant and presents a great variability. Having the elbow extended and the forearm fully supinated, the radial artery is found medially from the DBT at its origin from the brachial artery, and there is at least one radial recurrent artery always, which crosses more proximal and volar the DBT than the radial artery. The main artery pattern consists of a single radial recurrent artery (RRA), which derives from the radial artery and crosses superficially on the tendon at 4 mm proximal and 15.4 mm volar to the most proximal site of the tuberosity. This artery may bifurcate or trifurcate, and it may derive from the brachial or ulnar artery and up to three RRAs may be present and volar to the tendon.

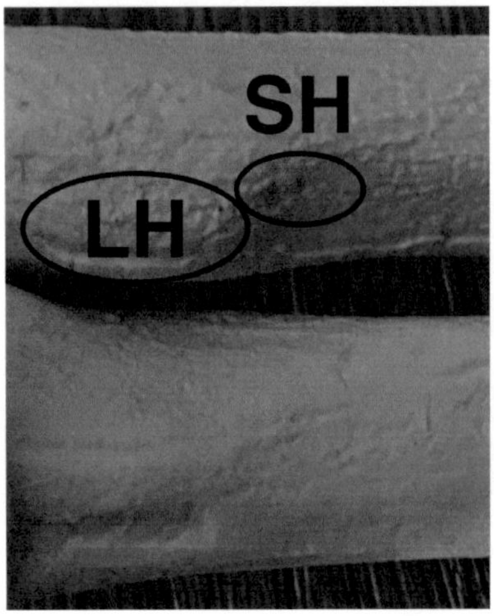

Figure 2.
Distal biceps footprint.

Both volarly and dorsally of the tendon, RRA may be encountered. In the same study, in 8 out of 17 specimens, a smaller RRA traversing dorsally the DBT was found on average 16 mm proximal to the volar RRA. On average, three veins cross volarly the DBT at 0.2 mm proximally and 16 mm volarly of the most proximal site of the radial tuberosity, and in general, they are found superficially to the arteries. In conclusion, when trying to repair a ruptured biceps tendon, three to six vascular structures might be encountered, and one should keep in mind that the rupture might alter their expected anatomic relations (**Figure 3**) [9].

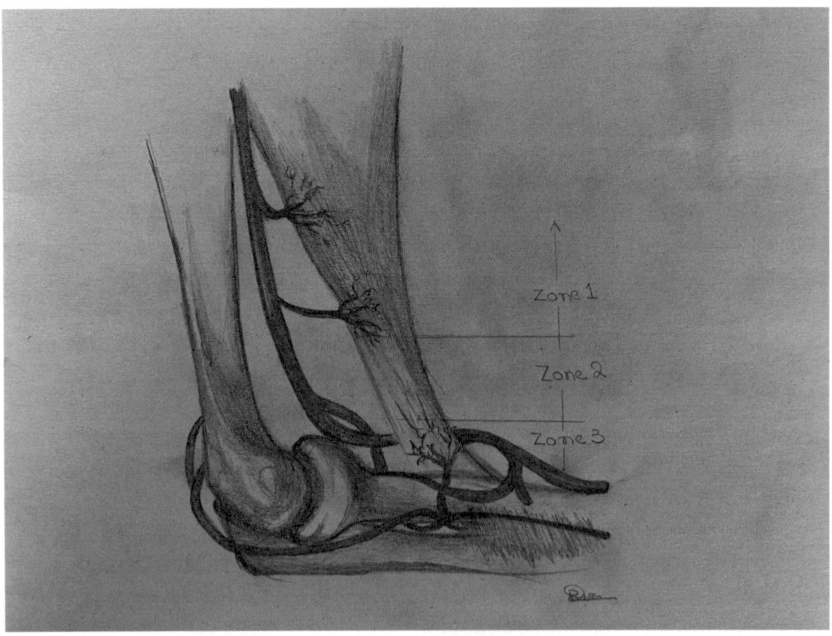

Figure 3.
Vascular anatomy.

1.2 Diagnosis

1.2.1 Clinical diagnosis

The diagnosis of DBT rupture is mostly based on history and clinical examination. A sudden, painful, audible 'pop' is typically felt during the act of rupture when trying to lift a heavy object or with excessive eccentric contraction and abrupt elbow extension [2]. Painful resisted elbow flexion and forearm supination are usually evident, along with a decrease in strength. The 'Popeye sign' is often noted due to superior migration of the muscle belly, and a palpable gap can be felt. Ecchymosis is commonly seen in the antecubital fossa and the medial aspect of the elbow a few days from injury.

The biceps squeeze test, and the hook test can be utilized to diagnose a complete tendon rupture, both tests having a sensitivity of 100% and specificity of 95 and 100%, respectively. The hook test is performed, having the elbow at 90° of flexion and the forearm supinated. The examiner then can hook his finger under the DBT from the lateral to medial direction when the tendon is intact or partially torn. In cases of DBT rupture, there is no cord-like structure that can be hooked under the finger, and that can be further confirmed by performing the test on the contralateral side [10]. The biceps squeeze test is utilized, having the elbow flexed at 60–80° and slightly pronated. Then, by squeezing the biceps muscle, supination of the forearm is noted normally, while in the case of ruptured DBT, there is no forearm movement [11]. The supination-pronation test is a reliable and painless exam where the examiner notes the change of shape of the biceps muscle belly while rotating the forearm. With DBT intact, elongation of the muscle belly at pronation should be recorded while the muscle is moving proximally at supination. Another specific test based on anatomic landmarks relies on measuring the interval between the antecubital fossa crease and the cusp of distal descent of the biceps muscle. The test is positive for DBT rupture with the sensitivity of 96% when the antecubital crease interval is higher than 6 cm or with a biceps crease interval ratio of more than 1.2 between the affected and non-affected arm [12].

When those tests are negative, the differential diagnosis includes primarily biceps tendonitis or partial tendon tears in an acute setting or in the ground of chronic degenerative tendinopathy. Those conditions mimic a complete biceps tendon tear as they present pain in resisted flexion of the elbow and supination of the forearm. Patients with partial DBT ruptures often present pain on deep palpation of the tendon in the antecubital fossa. The Distal biceps provocation test seems also reliable in the diagnosis of partial DBT tears. Pain at resisted elbow flexion of 70°, which is significantly higher in pronation than in supination, indicates a positive test and high reliability has been proposed for this test [13]. A strong indicator of insertional tendinopathy is when pain is elicited on palpation of the radial tuberosity on the posterolateral aspect of the elbow with the forearm pronated. As with every other tendon, same with biceps tendon, degeneration at the insertion site is frequent and although it may be asymptomatic, it is often recorded when surgically treating biceps ruptures. Other pathologies that may mimic a biceps tendon rupture include lateral elbow epicondylitis, plica syndrome and elbow arthritis.

1.2.2 Diagnostic images

Plain radiographic studies are of paramount importance in excluding other etiologies, but they do not provide any information when it comes to diagnosing a biceps tendon rupture. MRI survey can also be proved helpful in the differential diagnosis, especially when partial rupture is encountered, with a specific protocol [flexed elbow, abducted shoulder, forearm supinated (FABS) view], having on a prone patient the shoulder abducted at 180°, the elbow flexed at 90° and the forearm supinated [14]. When interpreting an MRI, the sign of a fluid-fill insertion site is compatible with complete rupture while high signal intensity, thinning or thickening of the tendon through the course might correspond to a partial tear or tendonitis [14]. Ultrasound study is another modality that can be used, with the benefit of a low-cost and fast examination, although it lacks accuracy in comparison with MRI, and it is a user-dependent method [2].

1.3 Pathophysiology

The pathogenesis of DBT rupture includes blood supply insufficient segments as well as attritional syndrome of the tendon's fibers during pronotion – supination of the forearm. The proximal one-third and the distal one-third of the DBT have their own dedicated intratendinous blood supply from branches of the brachial artery and the posterior recurrent artery, respectively, whereas the hypovascular zone between them is supplied only in an extratendinous fashion from the paratendon [15]. It was also noted that even this extratendinous blood supply was decreased in the middle third with fewer and smaller vessels, while degenerative changes of the tendon's substance are also present in this area [15]. The same findings are presented by Koch et al.; a hypovascular area is found in the radial side of DBT where the tendon opposes the radius and presents a fibrocartilage structure, just above the insertion site [8].

The space between the lateral cortical margin of the ulna and the radial tuberosity is shortened to nearly 50% from supination to pronation not only because of the radius rotating over ulna but also as the distal ulna moves laterally creating an abduction moment of the ulna. DBT occupies roughly 85% of the radioulnar space at the level of the tuberosity during pronation and a prominent bicipital tuberosity ridge may contribute to an impingement syndrome [4, 15]. Bicipital tuberosity ridge might act as a knife-like margin as DBT glides over it before its final attachment during pronation of the forearm. This hypothesis is further enhanced by the fact that there has never been reported a DBT rupture on a patient with a smooth (no ridge) tuberosity [4]. In line with the aforementioned, using a quantitative 3D CT technique, Hilgersorm et al. have shown that radial tuberosity volume and height were maximum in patients who suffered from DBT rupture than in the control-healthy group [3]. So, apart from tensile forces, DBT is subjected to pressure and shearing forces that may render the tendon vulnerable to rupture [8]. Those two parameters (vascular and impingement) may predispose to a poor regeneration response of the tendon in degenerative and inflammatory changes in the segment just proximal to the enthesis that ultimately lead to rupture.

In terms of structural biology, two fibrocartilaginous parts of DBT have been identified: the first is in its insertion and the other is in the radial-gliding side of the tendon that abuts the radius during pronation. The gliding part of the DBT differs from the ulnar side DBT, which resembles a traction tendon. These differences include a rounded rather than an elongated cellular morphology, extracellular matrix and collagen fibers organization, and they are guided by the prevailing biomechanical conditions of this area of conflict [8]. The transition spot from fibrocartilaginous gliding tendon to a normal traction tendon is assumed to be susceptible to rupture after tensile force is applied, as it represents an area with different mechanical properties.

The lacertus fibrosus has been proposed as an etiological factor in biceps tendon rupture. Being a fixed-length structure, it is under tension during contraction of forearm flexor muscles and this imposed a medially oriented force onto the DBT in a manner that may contribute to the pathogenesis of rupture [5].

2. Surgical treatment of biceps tendon tears

2.1 Acute complete tears

It is widely recognized that surgical intervention enhances the strength of supination and flexion, along with improving fatigue resistance in both movements and maintaining a normal posture during full supination. Adequate supination strength is essential for tasks such as loosening a stuck bolt, swinging sports equipment like bats or golf clubs, and stabilizing tools effectively. However, there are specific contraindications to surgical reconstruction, including low functional demands, severe limitations in passive motion of the elbow and forearm, active infections, significant medical comorbidities, and a compromised soft tissue envelope.

Morrey et al. first documented an average reduction of 40% in supination strength and a 30% decrease in flexion strength following nonoperative intervention. It is significant to highlight that prompt reattachment led to the restoration of normal flexion and supination strength, while delayed reinsertion enhanced both flexion and supination strength, albeit not completely returning it to baseline levels [16].

The initial effort to attach the distal biceps tendon to the radial tuberosity was documented in 1898, whereas the first recorded reinsertion using a device, specifically a nail, occurred in 1928 [17].

Currently, there are three primary debates surrounding surgical repair techniques: the choice between single and double-incision exposure, between anatomical and non-anatomical repair, and the preferred fixation method (most commonly the use of cortical button, interference screws, transosseous sutures or suture anchors) [18].

2.1.1 Single-incision approach

2.1.1.1 Cortical button technique

This technique, first described by Bain et al. in the early 2000s, involves a single anterior incision that facilitates an anatomical repair [19]. A 5-cm transverse skin incision is executed approximately 2 cm distal to the elbow skin crease, followed by identification of the lateral antebrachial cutaneous nerve. Within the bursa, the retracted biceps tendon is readily identified. In cases of acute injury, the tendon tract can be easily located as it extends toward the radial tuberosity. With the elbow fully extended and supinated, exposure of the radial tuberosity is achieved using retractors. A cortical window sufficient for accommodating the tendon is created with a high-speed burr; it is crucial for this window to be positioned as medially as possible in a fully supinated forearm to ensure proper fixation of the tendon at its anatomical insertion point.

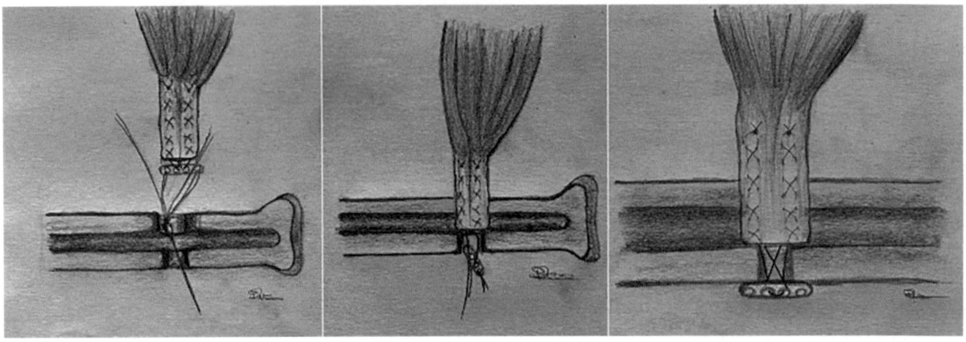

Figure 4.
Single incision cortical button.

A drill equipped with a guard is inserted into the cortical window to create a hole in the posterior cortex, facilitating passage for the button. The preparation of the radial tuberosity can be efficiently conducted while keeping both elbow and forearm in their respective positions—full extension and supination (**Figure 4**).

The retracted distal segment of the biceps tendon is extracted outside of the wound for debridement of any necrotic tissue at its end. A non-absorbable suture (number 5 Ethibond) secures this tendon to two central holes within the button, while Bunnell sutures are incorporated into both medial and lateral edges of the tendon with knots positioned proximally. It is essential to maintain an approximate gap of 2 mm between the button and free tendon end to facilitate manipulation through the dorsal cortex of the radius; this space may require adjustment based on radius size. Knots are secured proximally allowing potential retightening if it was necessary.

For suture placement, a non-absorbable (number 1 Ethibond) suture enters through one leading hole of the endobutton, while a trailing hole accommodates a non-absorbable suture (1/O Prolene); both are threaded onto an elongated straight-eyed needle. In a supinated position, this needle traverses through both cortical window and drill hole exiting *via* posterior forearm skin. To ensure safety from injury to surrounding nerves, particularly avoiding contact with the posterior interosseous nerve (PIN), an ulnar direction during insertion is adopted. Numerous cadaveric studies in the literature indicate a particular direction for button placement to prevent injury to the posterior interosseous nerve (PIN). Most evidence supports an orientation of either 30 degrees proximally, 30 degrees ulnarly, or a combination of both [20, 21].

Upon applying tension on the lead suture (number 1 Ethibond), both button and trailing tendon are guided into place within cortical window without twisting or excessive tensioning. Flexion of elbow aids in ensuring that Endobutton successfully exits at opposite cortex location. Once through, radius completion occurs by applying tension on trailing Prolene suture, guaranteeing locking within subperiosteal space situated on dorsal side of radius.

Fluoroscopy provides critical oversight regarding Endobutton positioning during advancement across radius structure. The elbow undergoes full range motion assessment confirming secure attachment of biceps tendon distal aspect remains within medullary canal correlating with radial tuberosity level before finally removing number 1 Ethibond and Prolene sutures (**Figure 5**).

DOI: http://dx.doi.org/10.5772/intechopen.1009204

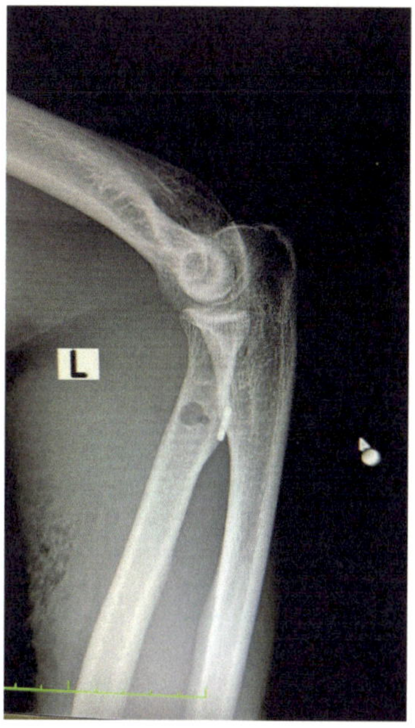

Figure 5.
Single incision cortical button.

2.1.1.2 Tension slide: Button technique

This method represents a modification of the cortical button technique initially introduced by Bain et al. [19]. A significant challenge associated with the conventional cortical button technique is the necessity for the surgeon to accurately estimate the length of the suture connecting the button to the biceps tendon, which often leads to inaccuracies. During cyclical loading of the construct between bone and button, even a minor displacement of 3 mm can result in a full 1 cm separation. This gap between the bone and tendon may compromise both the strength and subsequent healing process of the tendon. In response to this issue, Sethi and Tibone proposed the Tension Slide technique in 2008 as a potential solution [22].

A 4-cm transverse incision is made approximately 4 cm distal to the elbow flexion crease. The lateral antebrachial cutaneous nerve is located and retracted laterally. The distal segment of the biceps tendon is exposed and subjected to minimal debridement. A No. 2 polyester suture is employed to secure the distal 2.5 cm of the biceps tendon using the Krakow suture technique.

Next, the suture is threaded through a button. The initial strand is passed through the right hole, and then returned through the left hole. Conversely, the other tail of the same suture is threaded through the left hole before being pulled back through the right hole. This results in both strands oriented toward the distal biceps tendon, with an approximate gap of 4 to 5 cm between the button and the end of the biceps tendon to facilitate manipulation through the radial tuberosity (**Figure 6**).

With the elbow held in full extension and supination, any remaining tissue on the radial tuberosity is debrided. A 3.2-mm guide pin is drilled through the center of this area from anterior to posterior. Following this, an 8.0-mm cannulated reamer enlarges both the anterior cortex and intramedullary canal to enable flush seating for the end of the distal biceps tendon.

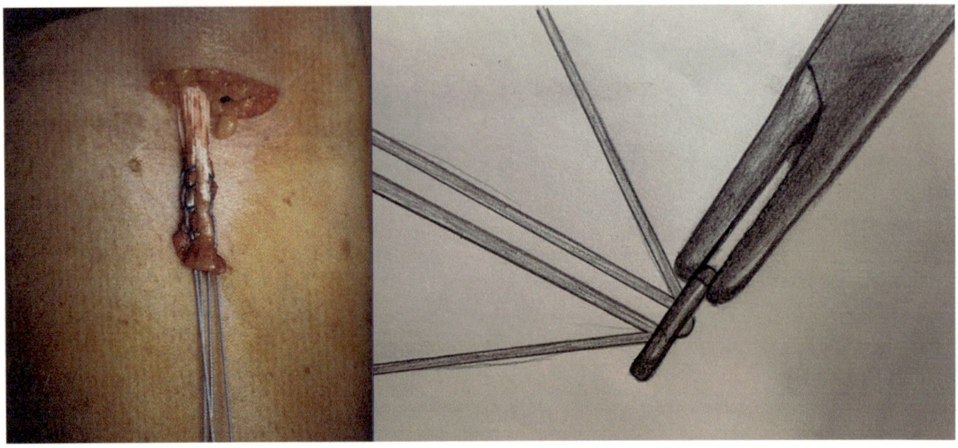

Figure 6.
Tension slide technique.

A button inserter or blunt end of a guide pin, which secures the button, assists in passing it through the tuberosity while minimizing potential nerve injury risks. Upon releasing it from its holder, tactile feedback confirms its positioning; fluoroscopy may be utilized for visualization at this stage.

To assess stability, tension is applied by pulling on each limb of suture separately; as one limb is gripped in each hand and gradually tightened, it facilitates docking of biceps into its prepared bone socket. Flexing at a range of 20 to 30 degrees aids in guiding tendon placement into position.

For patients with lower activity demands, a free needle can be used to pass one end of No. 2 polyester sutures through that portion of biceps tendon closest to its tuberosity and was tied. In contrast, for more active patients, insertion of a 7 by 10 mm interference screw on radial side occurs with additional tying of the suture limbs over the screw. Finally, it is essential to evaluate elbow motion across its full range to confirm the secure attachment of tendon.

2.1.1.3 Intramedullary cortical button fixation repair

Due to the risk of injury to the PIN nerve, Siebenlist et al. recommended using one or two intramedullary buttons to securely anchor the biceps tendon to the tuberosity (**Figure 7**) [23].

As previously outlined, an anterior incision is utilized to expose and prepare both the biceps tendon and the biceps tuberosity. The procedure for two intramedullary cortical button fixation is almost the same as single fixation. To facilitate the placement of these buttons within the intramedullary canal, a 3.2-mm drill is angled at 60° relative to the radial head, targeting only the anterior cortex. The initial drilling site is strategically located at the proximal edge of the tuberosity ridge on each specimen, ensuring uniform implantation. Following drilling, a button is introduced through the anterior cortex and subsequently flipped into position using a button inserter. To avoid interference between buttons within the medullary canal, a custom parallel drill guide featuring a defined spacing of 12 mm was employed. In cases of one intramedullary fixation, a single button is positioned at the center of the radial tuberosity ridge.

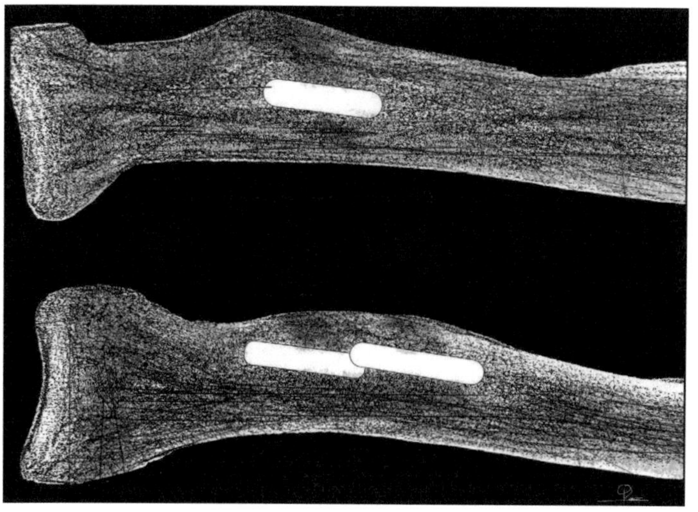

Figure 7.
Intramedullary technique.

2.1.1.4 Suture anchor fixation

The advancement and implementation of anchors in orthopedics have also facilitated their application in the treatment of distal biceps ruptures. Initial descriptions of the use of anchors for the repair of biceps ruptures were published in the early 2000s. We will outline the technique presented by Goljan et al. in 2016 [24], which is the same technique that we use.

An incision measuring approximately 6 cm is made on the anterior aspect of the skin, positioned just below the elbow flexion crease and medial to the mobile wad. The lateral antebrachial cutaneous nerve is identified and retracted laterally. In acute cases, the torn biceps tendon is typically found superficially within the antecubital fossa. Conversely, in delayed presentations, the distal portion of the tendon may retract more proximally above the elbow crease. Upon locating the distal tendon stump, it is debrided until healthy tissue is visible. A stay suture is then placed to facilitate traction, while adhesions between the tendon and biceps muscle belly are released to maximize tendon mobility.

With the forearm fully supinated, exposure of the radial tuberosity is achieved while protecting the posterior interosseous nerve. Careful placement of retractors around the proximal radius enhances visibility during this procedure. Any remaining tendon remnants are excised, and the bicipital tuberosity is curetted down to bleeding bone. Two anchors equipped with non-absorbable sutures (No. 2 Ethibond) are inserted both proximally and distally into the bicipital tuberosity, ensuring a minimum 1-cm bone bridge between them. Fluoroscopy aids in verifying their correct placement, followed by extensive irrigation of the area to eliminate any bone debris.

Distal traction is applied to the tendon, ensuring it has sufficient mobility while allowing it to move closer to the bicipital tuberosity during elbow flexion. Once the tendon exhibits an adequate range of motion, fixation with sutures is carried out. The suture limbs from each anchor are maneuvered within their respective anchors, which facilitates smooth advancement of the suture – a critical aspect of this technique as

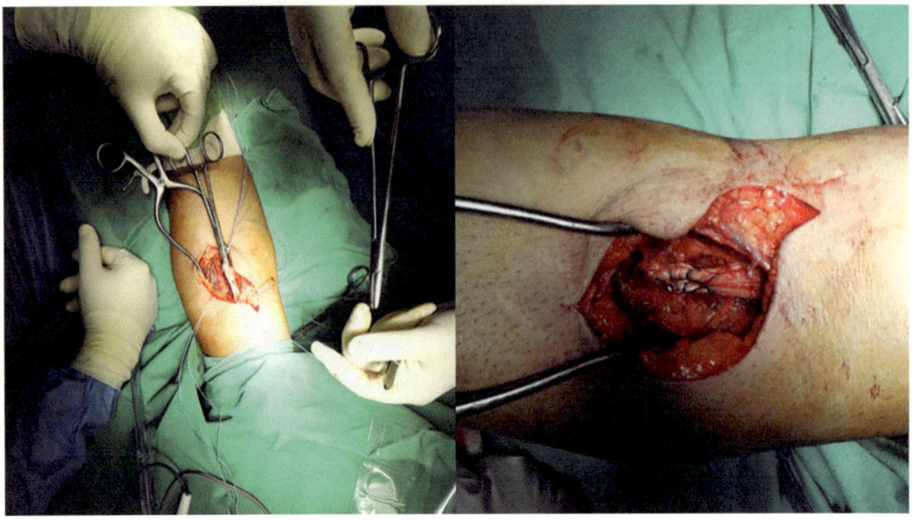

Figure 8.
Single anchors.

it enables proper alignment of the tendon at its insertion point. After confirming the mobility of the sutures, both anchor limbs are positioned such that one limb measures two-thirds the total length of the suture. This longer limb is utilized for fixing the tendon, while the shorter limb serves to apply tension.

The longer suture limb of the proximal anchor is threaded through the medial aspect of the tendon, starting roughly 5 mm from the edge. Three running-locking (Krakow) stitches are executed, with each stitch spaced 8 to 10 mm apart, ensuring that the final stitch emerges from a deep position to rest on top of the tendon. Subsequently, the shorter suture limb of this same anchor is inserted through the tendon in a deep-to-superficial direction, positioned about 5 mm from the distal tendon's end and situated between the running suture and the midpoint of the tendon. At this stage, these sutures are clamped while fixation is performed using the other anchor (**Figure 8**).

With the same technique, the extended suture from the second, more distal anchor is threaded through the outermost part of the tendon, positioned 2 to 3 mm away from its edge. Three Krakow sutures are then implemented, with the suture limb remaining on the top of the tendon. Then, the shorter limb of this distal second anchor is passed in a deep-to-superficial manner through the center of the tendon, approximately 5 mm from its distal edge. With the arm fully supinated and flexed at 90 degrees, tension is applied to the "shorter" limb of the proximal anchor, effectively drawing the biceps tendon down toward the tuberosity. The two sutures from this proximal anchor are tied together to secure the tendon to bone. Finally, both limbs of the distal anchor are tied together to ensure adequate fixation and restore the insertional footprint.

2.1.1.5 Bioabsorbable interference screw fixation

Bioabsorbable interference screw fixation has gained significant regard, particularly in operations around the knee. Numerous studies have assessed the biomechanical characteristics of these screws.

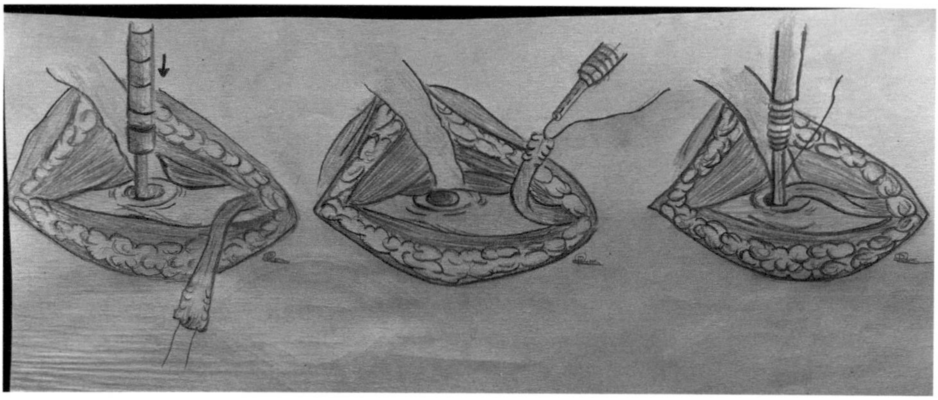

Figure 9.
Bioabsorbable screw fixation.

According to Mazzocca et al. [25], this technique represents an adaptation of the anterior longitudinal Henry approach. During the procedure, the lateral antebrachial cutaneous nerve is identified and retracted laterally. The muscular interval between the pronator teres and brachioradialis is carefully developed bluntly until reaching the lacertus fibrosis.

Depending on the duration of the tear, the biceps tendon often retracts from the tuberosity, resulting in a bulbous appearance at its end. If the tendon exhibits fraying and degenerative collagen changes, we can remove at least 1 cm without any risk. A no. 2 Fiberwire (Arthrex, Inc., Naples, FL) is subsequently threaded using either a Krakow or whipstitch technique to the tendon for a distance of 12 to 13 mm proximally.

To ensure optimal visualization of the tuberosity, the arm should be positioned in maximal supination and extension. The tuberosity typically has a fibrous layer of immature scar tissue that must be excised for clear visualization. A guide pin is inserted into the center of the tuberosity, followed by an 8 mm reamer to create an 8-mm hole through just the proximal cortex (**Figure 9**).

The tenodesis driver is composed of a cannulated handle and a post. After positioning the selected screw onto the driver, sutures from the distal end of the prepared tendon can be threaded through it. The post facilitates the insertion of the tendon into the base of the socket and secures it while an interference screw is advanced over it using a threaded mechanism. To execute the tenodesis, one end of the Fiberwire suture is threaded through the tenodesis driver along with an attached 8 × 12 mm screw. The driver is then inserted into an 8-mm hole, ensuring that the tendon is situated on the ulnar aspect of the tuberosity. With stabilization provided by Addson forceps, the screw is advanced through the tenodesis driver as previously described. Once the screw has been fully inserted and the tenodesis driver has been withdrawn, the suture passing through the cannulated screw is secured to the exterior of the interference screw.

2.1.1.6 A single posterior incision approach with sutures

Kelly et al. introduced an innovative posterior incision technique for addressing partial ruptures of the biceps tendon [26]. This approach facilitates direct access to the radial tuberosity, where the partially torn tendon remains connected. It would be feasible to

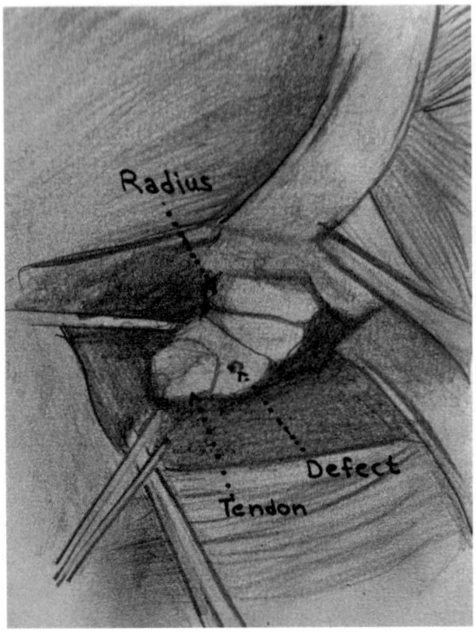

Figure 10.
Posterior incision approach.

examine and securely reattach the biceps tendon to the radial tuberosity through a single posterior skin incision without the risks of anterior incision (**Figure 10**).

The radial tuberosity can be identified by palpating the lateral forearm while it is fully pronated or by measuring downward from the olecranon on a lateral preoperative radiograph. A 4-cm incision is subsequently made, positioned directly over the radial tuberosity, approximately 1 cm anterolateral to the ulna's subcutaneous border. The fascia of the extensor digitorum communis is then split longitudinally in alignment with the skin incision. For posterior interosseous nerve protection, the forearm should remain in full pronation while longitudinally splitting the supinator fascia over the radial tuberosity, which allows for visualization of the underlying biceps tendon at its radius insertion.

With the forearm fully pronated, any residual tendon fibers on the radial tuberosity are removed. Maintaining this full pronation, a large burr is employed to form a bone trough measuring 6 to 8 mm in width and 10 mm in length within the radial tuberosity. A cavity is then excavated to expose the medullary canal of the proximal radius, thereby creating an area for the tendon to be seated. Subsequently, three drill holes are made, spaced 7 to 8 mm apart and positioned 7 to 10 mm from the edge of the trough while keeping the arm in slight pronation.

Two non-absorbable sutures (No. 2 Ethibond) are intricately threaded through the tendon in a Krakow technique, creating four distinct strands. These suture strands are then passed through the bone trough and out of the drilled holes – one strand exiting each of the proximal and distal openings and two strands emerging from the central hole. The tendon is subsequently retracted into the bone trough by supinating the forearm and exerting tension on the sutures, which are ultimately secured over the bone bridges.

3. Dual-incision approach

The benefit of the two-incision technique lies in its ability to facilitate a more posterior attachment of the biceps to the radial tuberosity. This approach not only restores anatomical integrity but also enhances the biomechanical advantage of supination.

3.1 Bone tunnels with sutures

The dual-incision technique was first described in 1960 by Meherin et al. [27], involving a cohort of only six patients in whom the biceps tendon was reattached to the radial tuberosity. Subsequently, Boyd and Anderson popularized this two-incision approach to mitigate the risk of iatrogenic injury to the posterior interosseous nerve (PIN) [28]. A primary advantage of this technique is its capacity to achieve a more anatomical restoration of the native footprint of the distal biceps tendon. Morrey and colleagues later modified the technique to minimize the risk of radioulnar synostosis by employing a muscle-splitting approach [29].

A standard two-incision, muscle-splitting method is utilized for the double-incision bone tunnel technique. The tendon is prepared using a conventional locking whipstitch. Identification of the radial tuberosity is performed *via* the dorsal approach, followed by debridement of any biceps tendon remnants. A high-speed burr is meticulously employed to create a trough measuring approximately 8 mm in width and 10 mm in length, ensuring that the trough constitutes less than 30% of the overall diameter to prevent it from becoming a stress riser and a potential site for fracture.

Upon preparation of the trough, two drill holes are created and positioned proximal and/or lateral to the trough. A passing suture is then threaded through each drill hole for the subsequent passage of the free suture on the biceps tendon. The biceps tendon is subsequently positioned medially to the radius and retrieved through the posterior incision. The free ends of the biceps suture are shuttled through the drill holes and securely tied over a bone bridge (**Figure 11**) [30].

Furthermore, the original technique, as modified by Morrey et al., may also be employed. This variation entails running two separate whipstitches along the biceps tendon and utilizing three drill holes, with one suture from each whipstitch passing

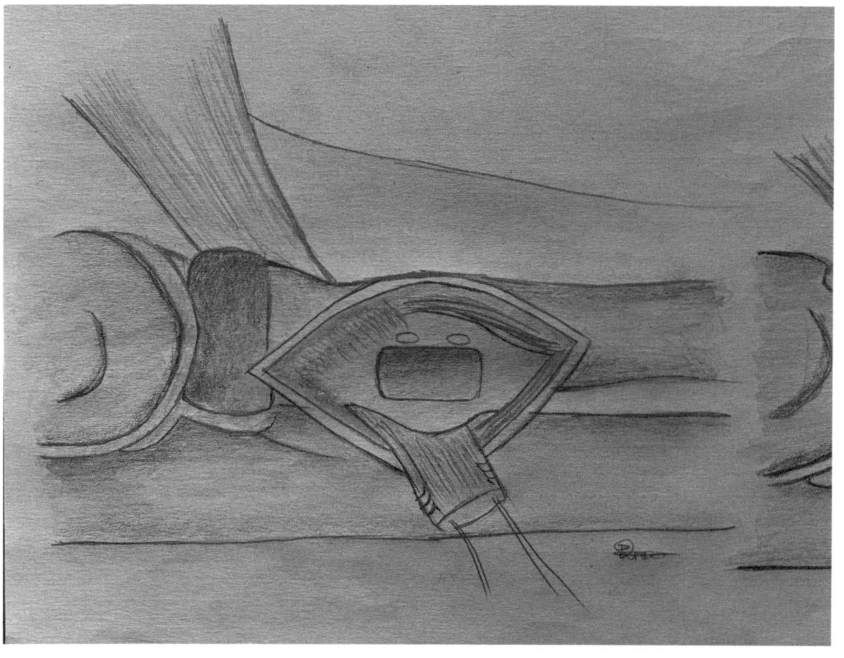

Figure 11.
Dual-incision technique with sutures.

through the proximal and distal drill holes, while the remaining two are threaded through the middle drill hole.

3.2 Unicortical buttons

Schmidt recommended a posterior incision measuring 3 to 4 cm over the extensor carpi ulnaris (ECU), aligned parallel to the ulna [31]. The incision is initiated 2 cm distal to the lateral epicondyle and 2.5 cm dorsal to the ulnar ridge. To mitigate the risk of injury to the radial nerve, the forearm should be pronated, allowing for dissection of the ECU muscle along its fibers to expose the obliquely oriented supinator muscle. The supinator muscle should be incised directly over the radial tuberosity, which can be palpated in the pronated forearm or located using intraoperative fluoroscopy. It is essential to clear the area of soft tissue surrounding the footprint.

Schmidt employed unicortical buttons for fixation. A 3.2 mm drill was utilized to create near-cortex holes at the center of the footprint for each head. To facilitate the flipping of the unicortical buttons within the medullary canal, the drill holes were angled at 60° distal to the radial shaft. Subsequently, with the forearm fully supinated, a Kelly clamp was used to guide the tendon from the anterior to the posterior aspect along its designated pathway. To maintain the tendon's normal orientation, it was externally rotated 90° and passed along this trajectory, ensuring that the short head (solid color) inserts distally and the long head (striped color) inserts proximally on the footprint. The docking limb of each suture was threaded through the central holes of the cortical button and into their respective drill holes (short: distal, long: proximal) (**Figure 12**). The buttons were seated against the near cortex by applying pressure with the flat end of the drill pin and pulling on the docking suture arm. Traction on the docking limbs of each suture compresses the corresponding biceps heads against the footprint. Prior to securing the sutures, fluoroscopy may be employed to confirm that both buttons

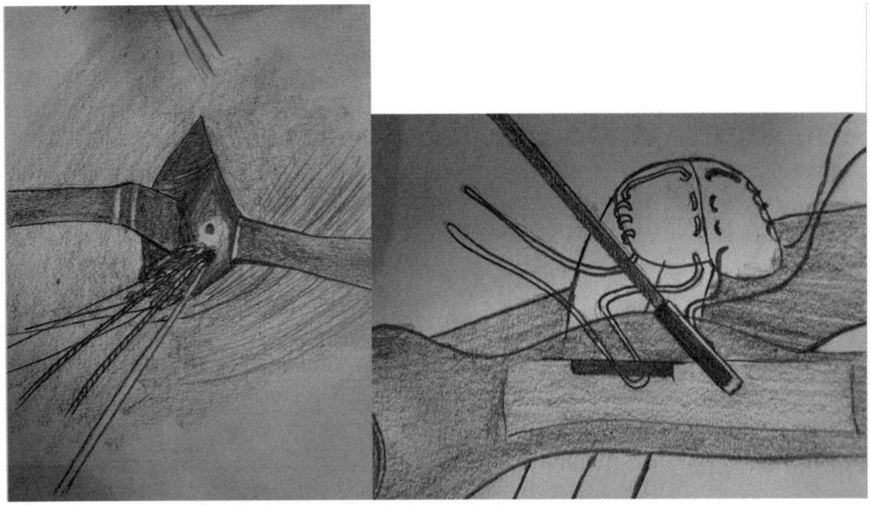

Figure 12.
Unicortical technique.

are properly seated parallel to and in contact with the near cortex. Each button subsequently functions as an intramedullary pulley, and the repair is finalized by tying multiple knots to secure it.

4. Endoscopic technique

The endoscopic technique for distal biceps repair was first introduced by Eames et al. for the management of partial ruptures of the tendon; however, it is now also employed for the repair of complete ruptures of the biceps tendon.

In 2006, Eames et al. detailed the surgical procedure, the elbow crease is identified by flexing the elbow, after which a 2 cm incision is made 3 cm distal to the elbow crease, centrally on the forearm [32]. Throughout the procedure, the lateral antebrachial cutaneous nerve is identified and protected. In the case of a partial tear, the tendon is palpated and traced to its insertion point. Retractors are utilized throughout the procedure to minimize the risk of damaging the anterior neurovascular structures. A small portal is created in the bicipital bursa, which can be accomplished either by sharp dissection or by piercing it with a trocar. The endoscope is then positioned between the tendon and the bicipital tuberosity to evaluate the extent of the tear. In instances of fraying of the tendon, visibility may be compromised.

A shaver is introduced to facilitate debridement, which is best achieved by opening the mouth of the shaver and placing it on the cannula of the endoscope, allowing it to glide to the tip of the scope. The tendon is debrided until a clear view of the tear is obtained. An algorithm has been developed to guide subsequent treatment. If there is no tear but inflammation of the tendon and bursa is observed, the bursa is excised. This can be performed under direct visualization through the portal or as an arthroscopic technique using the shaver, depending on the surgeon's preference.

For partial tears involving less than 25% of the tendon width, debridement of the tear is performed. If the tear encompasses between 25 and 50% of the insertion, the tendon is debrided and reinserted using a bone anchor. In cases where the tear involves more than 50% of the insertion, the entire tendon is released and reinserted using the button technique for fixation.

The approach differs somewhat in acute tears with tendon retraction. In such cases, the tuberosity is palpated and approached *via* blunt dissection. The endoscope provides a direct view of the tuberosity, allowing for debridement of the footprint at this stage. The scope can then be utilized to trace the path of the retracted biceps until the tendon stump is visualized. Flexing the elbow may assist in locating the stump. A clamp is then applied to the tendon, which is pulled through the skin for reinsertion according to the surgeon's preference. The endoscope is employed to identify the correct position and placement of the guide pin. Once the appropriate position is confirmed, the endoscopic technique follows the same protocol as the mini-open button fixation technique.

In 2009, Gregory et al. also described an endoscopic surgical technique utilizing suture anchors for tendon stabilization [33]. A 3-cm incision is made in the "safe area," located in the medial aspect of the transverse anterior elbow crease, just proximal to the convergence of the distal biceps brachii tendon, with the surrounding neurovascular structures situated distal to this area. The tendon sheath is identified and longitudinally incised for the evacuation of hematoma and saline lavage of the tendon tract to prevent heterotrophic ossification. The retracted proximal end of the tendon is grasped from within the proximal sheath using a clip and pulled out through the portal. The ruptured tendon end is then freshened, while ensuring the lateral cutaneous nerve of the forearm is identified and protected, as it may come into contact with the bicipital aponeurosis.

Next, with the elbow flexed and the forearm in supination, the endoscopic sheath is introduced into the distal tendon tract up to the radial tuberosity, followed by the insertion of a 4.5-mm endoscope in air (without fluid) positioned in flexion and supination. Prior to the insertion of the endoscope, the tendon sheath is properly cleaned with a sterile pad. The absence of soft tissue interposition and the correct positioning of the planned reinsertion area on the radial tuberosity are verified. An anchor is then inserted into the radial tuberosity, and the distal end of the tendon is brought out through the surgical incision. One limb of the suture anchor is passed through the distal 2 to 4 cm of the tendon and reinforced using a modified Kessler stitch technique. As the knot is tied, the tendon is pulled down and secured to the floor of the radial tuberosity, ensuring that the forearm is in maximum supination.

5. Chronic ruptures

Patients who seek treatment later for a distal biceps rupture typically fall into two categories: those whose initial diagnosis was overlooked and those who continue to experience pain and functional limitations despite an initial conservative treatment approach [18].

Several complications arise when managing chronic tears surgically. Within just a few weeks, the muscle and tendon retract proximally, lose their elasticity, and undergo atrophy [34]. Moreover, the natural canal through which the biceps tendon passes becomes filled with fibrous tissue, making reconstruction challenging. Additionally, the lateral antebrachial cutaneous nerve may become adhered to the muscle belly, necessitating more extensive dissection of the nerve, which could result in a higher incidence of postoperative nerve dysfunction.

Traditionally, it has been believed that most chronic distal biceps tendon (DBT) tears necessitate some type of augmentation during surgical intervention. This perspective largely stemmed from the observation that following the primary repair of chronic tears, retraction often resulted in severely restricted elbow extension at the conclusion of the procedure. Consequently, surgeons harbored concerns regarding the potential for permanent loss of elbow extension or the risk of re-rupture.

Recent evidence, however, indicates that a significant number of chronic tears can be addressed primarily, even in instances where elbow extension remains limited post-surgery. Patients appear capable of stretching their biceps and achieving a satisfactory range of motion without a concerning incidence of re-rupture [35]. This evolving understanding has led to modifications in our clinical practice.

Previously, the necessity for graft augmentation was determined exclusively based on the duration since injury. Currently, this decision is made intra-operatively; primary repair is preferred as long as sufficient tendinous tissue is available and the repair can be accomplished with the elbow flexed no more than 90 degrees. Repairing the DBT at higher degrees of flexion presents considerable challenges when utilizing a single-incision technique; conversely, employing transosseous sutures over

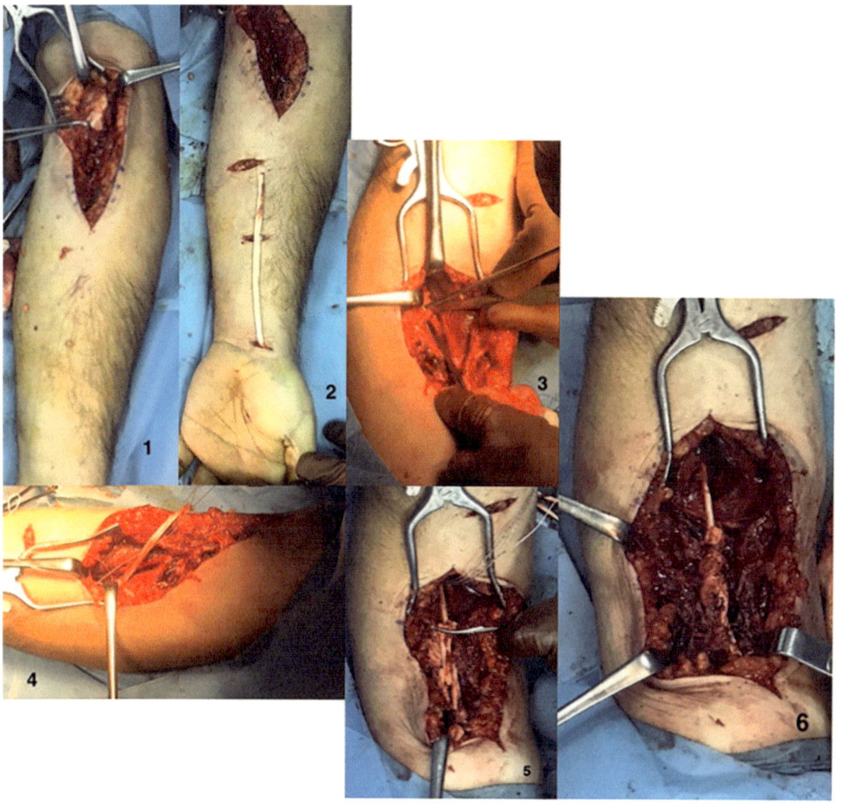

Figure 13.
Chronic ruptures.

the radius while accommodating any necessary degree of elbow flexion simplifies this process. Furthermore, as noted earlier, a preserved lacertus fibrosus serves as an excellent indicator for successfully performing a primary repair on chronic tears (**Figure 13**).

Graft augmentation is employed when there is a complete absence of tendon structure, particularly in instances of significant retraction [22]. Graft reconstruction may be carried out through either a single-incision or dual-incision approach, with various previously discussed methods available for securing the graft tendon to the radius. It is necessary to perform a more extensive anterior dissection proximally to adequately mobilize the biceps and selectively dissect the lateral antebrachial cutaneous nerve (LACB). The choice between autografts and allografts largely hinges on their availability and the preferences of the operating surgeon. Reconstruction techniques may involve utilizing interposing tendon autografts, such as semitendinosus, flexor carpi radialis, palmaris longus and hamstring tendons, or employing allografts from sources like Achilles, semitendinosus, and tibialis tendons [36]. Among these options, the semitendinosus autograft – capable of being interwoven into the distal biceps tendon (DBT) – and Achilles allograft are favored choices for chronic DBT tears. Initially, the Achilles allograft was applied with an attached calcaneal bone block to facilitate bone-to-bone integration at the bicipital tuberosity. Recent research has shown that excellent clinical and functional outcomes can be achieved using Achilles allografts without a calcaneal bone block [37].

6. Conclusion

The international literature highlights a variety of surgical techniques for the repair of distal biceps tendon ruptures. This chapter aims to elucidate the most significant of these techniques, particularly those that have marked pivotal advancements in the surgical restoration of biceps ruptures. Based on the existing literature, it is reasonable to conclude that the techniques described tend to yield favorable results in most patients. Surgeons should consider factors such as cost and their own level of experience when choosing between different methods.

Author details

Triantafyllos Katsimentzas[1*], Athina-Zacharoula Ditsiou[2], Vasileios Balamotis[3] and Konstantinos Ditsios[1]

1 2nd Orthopaedic Department, A.U.Th, Thessaloniki, Greece

2 A.U.Th, Thessaloniki, Greece

3 "Maillot" Hospital, Briey, France

*Address all correspondence to: triantafyllos_katsimentzas@hotmail.com

IntechOpen

© 2025 The Author(s). Licensee IntechOpen. This chapter is distributed under the terms of the Creative Commons Attribution License (http://creativecommons.org/licenses/by/4.0), which permits unrestricted use, distribution, and reproduction in any medium, provided the original work is properly cited.

References

[1] Safran MR, Graham SM. Distal biceps tendon ruptures: Incidence, demographics, and the effect of smoking. Clinical Orthopaedics and Related Research. 2002;**404**(404):275-283

[2] Jaschke M, Rekawek K, Sokolowski S, Kolodziej L. Distal biceps tendon rupture: A comprehensive overview. EFORT Open Reviews. 2023;**8**(11):865-873

[3] Hilgersom NFJ, Nagel M, Janssen SJ, Kodde IF, The B, Eygendaal D. Greater radial tuberosity size is associated with distal biceps tendon rupture: A quantitative 3-D CT case–control study. Knee Surgery, Sports Traumatology, Arthroscopy. 2021;**29**(12):4075-4081

[4] Mazzocca AD et al. The anatomy of the bicipital tuberosity and distal biceps tendon. Journal of Shoulder and Elbow Surgery. 2007;**16**(1):122-127

[5] Eames MHA, Bain GI, Fogg QA, Van Riet RP. Distal biceps tendon anatomy: A cadaveric study. Journal of Bone and Joint Surgery. 2007;**89**(5):1044-1049

[6] Athwal GS, Steinmann SP, Rispoli DM. The distal biceps tendon: Footprint and relevant clinical anatomy. The Journal of Hand Surgery. 2007;**32**(8):1225-1229

[7] Kulshreshtha R, Singh R, Sinha J, Hall S. Anatomy of the distal biceps brachii tendon and its clinical relevance. Clinical Orthopaedics and Related Research. 2007;**456**(456):117-120

[8] Koch S, Tillmann B. The distal tendon of the biceps brachii. Structure and clinical correlations. Annals of Anatomy. 1995;**177**(5):467-474

[9] Zeltser DW, Strauch RJ. Vascular anatomy relevant to distal biceps tendon repair. Journal of Shoulder and Elbow Surgery. 2016;**25**(2):283-288

[10] O'Driscoll SW, Goncalves LBJ, Dietz P. The hook test for distal biceps tendon avulsion. The American Journal of Sports Medicine. 2007;**35**(11):1865-1869

[11] Ruland RT, Dunbar RP, Bowen JD. The biceps squeeze test for diagnosis of distal biceps tendon ruptures. Clinical Orthopaedics and Related Research. 2005;**437**(437):128-131

[12] ElMaraghy A, Devereaux M, Tsoi K. The biceps crease interval for diagnosing complete distal biceps tendon ruptures. Clinical Orthopaedics and Related Research. 2008;**466**(9):2255-2262

[13] Caekebeke P, Schenkels E, Bell SN, van Riet R. Distal biceps provocation test. The Journal of Hand Surgery. 2021;**46**(8):710.e1-710.e4

[14] Giuffrè BM, Moss MJ. Optimal positioning for MRI of the distal biceps brachii tendon: Flexed abducted supinated view. American Journal of Roentgenology. 2004;**182**(4):944-946

[15] Seiler JG, Parker LM, Chamberland PDC, Sherbourne GM, Carpenter WA. The distal biceps tendon. Two potential mechanisms involved in its rupture: Arterial supply and mechanical impingement. Journal of Shoulder and Elbow Surgery. 1995;**4**(3):149-156

[16] Morrey BFA, Dobyns JH, An KN. Rupture of the distal tendon biceps brachii. A biomechanical study. Journal of Bone and Joint Surgery. 1985;**67**(3):418-421

[17] Dobbie RP. Avulsion of the lower biceps brachii tendon: Analysis of fifty-one previously unreported cases. American Journal of Surgery. 1941;**51**:662-683

[18] Alentorn-Geli E, Assenmacher AT, Sánchez-Sotelo J. Distal biceps tendon injuries: A clinically relevant current concepts review. EFORT Open Reviews. 2016;**1**(9):316-324

[19] Bain GI, Prem H, Heptinstall RJ, Verhellen R, Paix D. Repair of distal biceps tendon rupture: A new technique using the Endobutton. Journal of Shoulder and Elbow Surgery. 2000;**9**(2):120-126

[20] Saldua N, Carney J, Dewing C, Thompson M. The effect of drilling angle on posterior interosseous nerve safety during open and endoscopic anterior single-incision repair of the distal biceps tendon. Arthroscopy: The Journal of Arthroscopic & Related Surgery. 2008;**24**(3):305-310

[21] Mwaturura T, Peters MJ, Glaris Z, Goetz TJ. Safe drill trajectory for anatomic repair of distal biceps tendon through a single incision: A cadaveric study. The Journal of Hand Surgery. 2023;**48**(11):1160.e1-1160.e5

[22] Sethi PM, Tibone JE. Distal biceps repair using cortical button fixation. Sports Medicine and Arthroscopy Review. 2008;**16**(3):130-135

[23] Siebenlist S et al. Biomechanical *in vitro* validation of intramedullary cortical button fixation for distal biceps tendon repair: A new technique. The American Journal of Sports Medicine. 2011;**39**(8):1762-1768

[24] Goljan P, Patel N, Stull JD, Donnelly BP, Culp RW. Single incision distal biceps repair with hemi-Krackow suture technique: Surgical technique and early outcomes. The Hand. 2016;**11**(2):238-244

[25] Mazzocca AD, Alberta FG, Elattrache NS, Romeo AA. Single incision technique using an interference screw for the repair of distal biceps tendon ruptures. Operative Techniques in Sports Medicine. 2003;**11**(1):36-41

[26] Kelly EW, Steinmann S, O'Driscoll SW. Surgical treatment of partial distal biceps tendon ruptures through a single posterior incision. Journal of Shoulder and Elbow Surgery. 2003;**12**(5):456-461

[27] Meherin JM, Kilgore ES. The treatment of ruptures of the distal biceps brachii tendon. American Journal of Surgery. 1960;**99**(5):636-640

[28] Boyd HB, Anderson LD. A method for reinsertion of the distal biceps brachii tendon. Journal of Bone and Joint Surgery. 1961;**43**:1041-1043

[29] Kelly EW, Morrey BF, O'Driscoll. Complications of repair of the distal biceps tendon with the modified two-incision technique. Journal of Bone and Joint Surgery. 2000;**82**(11):575-581

[30] Savin DD et al. Surgical management of acute distal biceps tendon ruptures. Journal of Bone and Joint Surgery. 2017;**99**(9):785-796

[31] Schmidt CC, Styron JF, Lin EA, Brown BT. Distal biceps tendon anatomic repair. JBJS Essential Surgical Techniques. 2017;**7**(4):e32

[32] Eames MHA, Bain GI. Distal biceps tendon endoscopy and anterior elbow arthroscopy portal. Techniques in Shoulder & Elbow Surgery. 2006;**7**(3):139-142

[33] Grégory T, Roure P, Fontès D. Repair of distal biceps tendon rupture using a suture anchor: Description of a new endoscopic procedure. The American Journal of Sports Medicine. 2009;**37**(3):506-511

[34] Darlis NA, Sotereanos DG. Distal biceps tendon reconstruction in chronic ruptures. Journal of Shoulder and Elbow Surgery. 2006;**15**(5):614-619

[35] Srinivasan RC, Pederson WC, Morrey BF. Distal biceps tendon repair and reconstruction. The Journal of Hand Surgery. 2020;**45**(1):48-56

[36] Stoll LE, Huang JI. Surgical treatment of distal biceps ruptures. The Orthopedic Clinics of North America. 2016;**47**(1):189-205

[37] Snir N, Hamula M, Wolfson T, Meislin R, Strauss EJ, Jazrawi LM. Clinical outcomes after chronic distal biceps reconstruction with allografts. The American Journal of Sports Medicine. 2013;**41**(10):2288-2295

Section 3

Gynecological Obstetrical Surgery

Chapter 5

Surgical Techniques and Procedures in the Management of Postpartum Haemorrhage

Tripti Sinha

> *'Women are not dying because of a disease we cannot treat. They are dying because societies have yet to make the decision that their lives are worth saving.'*
>
> *Mahmoud F. Fathalla, President of the International Federation of Gynecology and Obstetrics (FIGO), World Congress, Copenhagen, 1997*

Abstract

Massive obstetric haemorrhage is a major cause of maternal mortality and near-miss and severe morbidity globally, especially in low-resource settings. Timely supportive measures and uterotonics and medications singly and in combination will salvage many lives. However, despite such measures, a significant number of cases continue to bleed. A natural corollary to this scenario is that all deliveries and complicated pregnancies should be managed in healthcare facilities with a 24x7 functional labour suite and operation theatre complex and/or swift transport facilities should referral be needed. Surgical interventions range from hysterectomy to uterus-conserving procedures. Uterine artery embolization requires a sophisticated setup not usually available in low-resource settings. Hence, obstetricians need to be conversant in a range of individualised surgical interventions which, if done at a proper stage in the management algorithm, can be lifesaving and often fertility preserving. Enhanced survival rates also mandate that obstetric ICU/HDU be organised in such obstetric facilities.

Keywords: stepwise devascularisation, antepartum haemorrhage, postpartum haemorrhage, obstetric hysterectomy, compression sutures

1. Introduction

Postpartum haemorrhage, romanticised by Taj Mahal built by Emperor Shah Jahan in memory of his queen Mumtaz Mahal who died in 1631 due to postpartum haemorrhage (PPH) following delivery of her fourteenth child, remains a nightmare and a management dilemma for any healthcare provider (HCP) attending deliveries [1]. The case of Mumtaz Mahal underscores PPH as a cause of maternal mortality and that high parity is an ominous risk factor. However, high parity should not detract the HCP from the sobering fact that PPH may occur in women of low parity including after the first delivery. Such cases underpin the reason why so many surgical techniques have evolved over time in an attempt to conserve the uterus and its fertility potential which is the focus of this chapter.

Despite rapid strides in maternity care, maternal mortality due to PPH remains alarming globally. Exact figures vary amongst countries, predominantly in low and middle-income countries (LMIC) and even in different regions of the same country determined mainly by the efficiency of the maternity services available to pregnant and labouring women there [2–4].

2. Basic considerations for rationale of surgical management of PPH

In order to understand the rationale of the various surgical techniques which have evolved over the years, it is important to understand the following aspects in relation to bleeding from the reproductive tract:

1. Cause of PPH: 4 Ts (Tone, Trauma, Tissue, Thrombin) (**Table 1**) [5]

2. Vascular supply of the reproductive tract (**Figure 1**)

2.1 Aetiology of postpartum haemorrhage

Table 1 summarises the aetiological causes of postpartum haemorrhage either singly or in combination.

2.2 Vascular supply of the uterus and pelvis

Figure 1 shows the vascular supply of the uterus. At term, blood flow to the uterus reaches 700 ml from 100 ml in the non-pregnant state.

In order to understand the rationale of the various surgical procedures which may be needed in management of PPH – conservative or uterine extirpative – the surgeon should be aware of the various vascular branches accessing the uterus including common variations encountered. The uterine corpus is chiefly supplied by the left and right uterine arteries, with some additional blood supply from branches of the ovarian arteries and collaterals from the upper vesical arteries. The lower uterine segment cervix and vagina derive their blood supply from the pelvic sub-epithelial collaterals arising from internal pudendal artery and accessory collaterals from internal iliac artery and lower vesical artery. Understanding the origin, distribution and anastomoses of the reproductive tract empowers the surgeon to decide which procedure is likely to work best in that particular case.

T	Clinical finding
Tone	uterine atony (multiple pregnancy, previous PPH, induced and/or augmented labor, prolonged first and second stage of labor, prolonged third stage, large fetus, distended bladder, general anaesthesia)
Trauma	uterine, cervical, vaginal or perineal injury, deep episiotomy, difficult instrumental delivery
Tissue	retained placenta or clots, placenta accreta
Thrombin	pre-existing or acquired coagulopathy (intra-uterine fetal demise, abruptio placentae, severe pregnancy induced hypertension)

Table 1.
Aetiology of PPH.

DOI: http://dx.doi.org/10.5772/intechopen.1010228

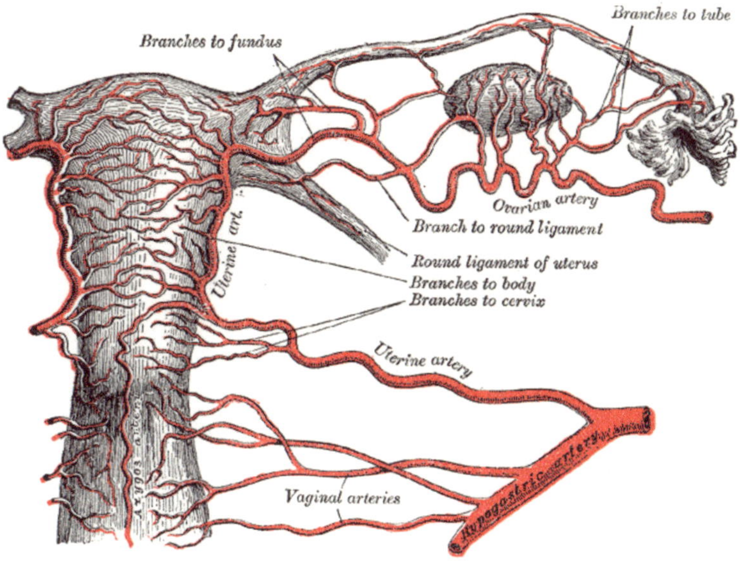

Figure 1.
Vascular supply of the uterus.

3. Management algorithm for PPH: The PPH care bundle

The management algorithm is based on the concept of 'golden hour', which is the vital time scale in which the decisions taken and the quality of care provided to the woman determines whether she survives the catastrophe or succumbs to the hypovolemic state with its lethal triad of hypothermia, coagulopathy and acidosis.

The first response to a case declared as having PPH is to call for '*HELP*'. This not only implies an increase in the number of HCPs summoned to assist in management but also may entail multi-disciplinary inputs with systematic co-ordinated strategies. Important decision points are embedded in the algorithm. The linked sequential steps in the management flowchart increase in complexity. Hence, the experience and competence in deciding performing procedures are essential attributes required of the HCP.

Table 1 and **Figure 2** are algorithms provided by the Ministry of Health and Family Welfare of Government of India. Its framework may be customised to adapt to local settings depending on resource availability.

3.1 The 20-minute rule

This is a guide in PPH emergencies to help HCPs attending PPH cases to decide how long they can persist with conservative measures before they step up the intervention to more aggressive steps.

1. First 20 minutes: IV fluids to combat hypovolemia, uterine massage, bimanual uterine compression, medical treatment (uterotonics, tranexamic acid), identification and management of cause keeping in mind the 4 Ts

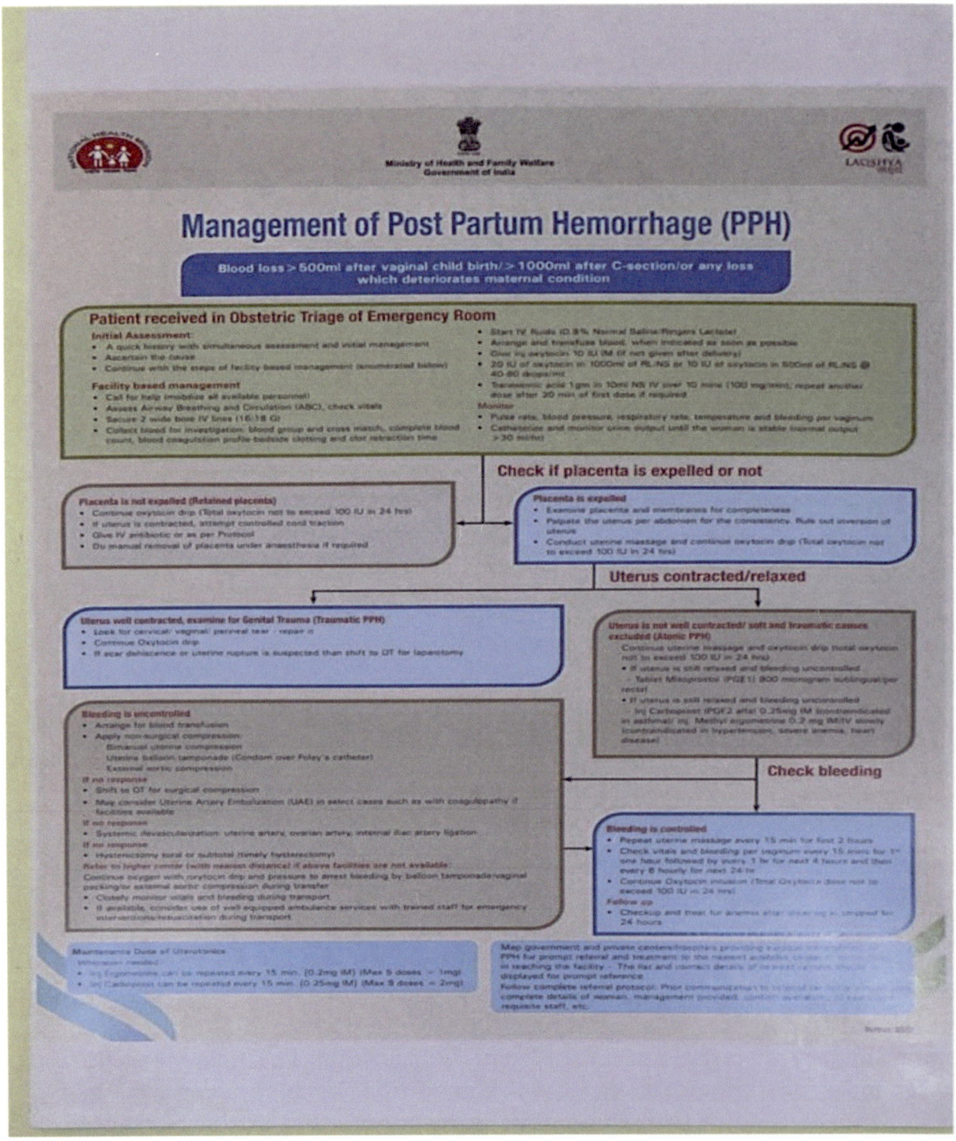

Figure 2.
Recommended flowchart for management of postpartum haemorrhage by Ministry of Health, Government of India.

2. Mechanical manoeuvres: intra-uterine balloon tamponade, uterine compression sutures (UCS), pelvic devascularisation procedures

3. Non-conservative surgery: hysterectomy, damage control surgery

PPH care bundle emphasises the multidisciplinary and co-ordinated team approach mandatory to effectively deliver care to woman having PPH. The care very often requires the woman to be referred and immediately transferred to a centre where more severity-appropriate care may be available. A robust transport ambulance with trained personnel very often makes the difference in terms of survival (**Figure 3**).

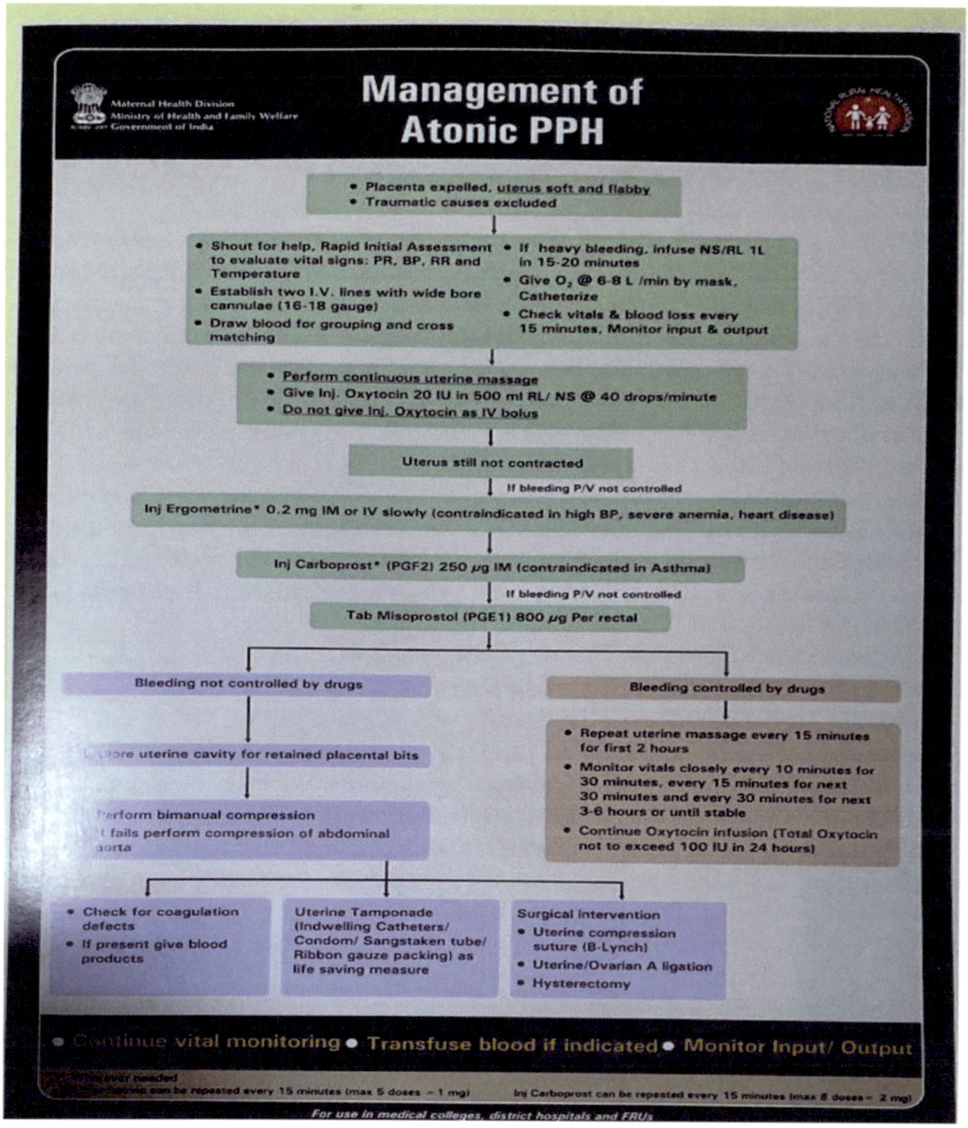

Figure 3.
Flowchart for management of atonic postpartum haemorrhage in low-resource settings(district hospitals and first referral units FRUs).

4. Role of surgery in atonic PPH

Traditionally, surgical interventions for PPH management included techniques depending on the cause identified. The decision to go ahead with the surgery is usually straightforward if the cause is retained tissue or injury anywhere in the reproductive tract. However, if the primary cause is atonic uterus or coagulopathy either de novo or a late feature of intractable PPH due to any other cause, the obstetrician is challenged on the following fronts:

1. At what stage in the patient management algorithm should one scale up the management to include surgical intervention/–s

2. Individualised choice of procedure: fertility sparing or uterine extirpation depending on the parity and future reproductive intentions of the woman.

3. Cause of bleeding

4. Topography of the bleeding site.

PPH secondary to uterine atony, placenta previa and placenta accreta syndrome (PAS) are the main challenges to the obstetric decision-making and surgical acumen. Although there are a variety of surgical procedures, each works only if done for the proper indication and in the proper manner. Each has its limitations and associated complications. It is incumbent on the surgeon to be fully conversant with all the above considerations related to the surgery chosen at that point of time. Procedure should have simplicity, safety and efficacy, efficacy being defined as the extent and rapidity with which the bleeding is controlled.

Figure 2 summarises the types of surgical procedures which have evolved over the years so that patients may survive the PPH as well as retain their fertility if that question arises. They range from pelvic vasculature occlusion methods and uterine compression sutures to the bleeding site to aggressive uterine extirpative procedures.

5. Emergency obstetric/peripartum hysterectomy (EOH/EPH)

Performing obstetric hysterectomy differs in several aspects from a routine hysterectomy performed for benign gynaecological indications. Gynaecological hysterectomy is usually performed as an elective procedure. The patient's general condition is optimised before she undergoes anaesthesia and surgery. Patient counselling also is done in settled calm settings where the patient and family have time to consider and consent for any management options explained to them. At operation also, the anatomy is less challenging with the ligaments, supports and vascular supply not grossly different from a non- pathological state.

All this changes when the need to perform obstetric hysterectomy arises out of the blue. Firstly, very often an anticipated straightforward vaginal or operative delivery goes grossly amiss. In such a circumstance, taking informed consent from the patient and her family itself is challenging– the care-providers and the patient with family are themselves stressed by the prior chain of events. Clear communication and documentation are mandatory to safeguard against medico-legal suits in future regardless of the outcome of the case.

Secondly, the anatomy and vascularity of the uterus and adnexa at term or near term are completely different from the non-pregnant state. At the uterine cornua, the round ligament, ovarian ligament and fallopian tubes do not converge but are spread out due to uterine myo-hyperplasia. The uterine circulation is extremely hyperdynamic, hence vascular pedicles are alarmingly broad. The demarcation between the uterine corpus, lower uterine segment (isthmus in non-pregnant state) and upper vagina is not distinct so it may be difficult to decide at what level the uterus may be truncated without reducing the vaginal length unnecessarily.

Indications for an obstetric hysterectomy include a badly ruptured uterus which cannot be repaired into a functional organ for subsequent child-bearing, uterine atony unresponsive to medical and other conservative measures, placenta accreta/percreta (morbidly adherent placenta), major degrees of placenta previa, severe puerperal genital sepsis or secondary PPH with adherent placental tissue difficult to remove in toto and which opens up large venous and arterial vessels in the bed.

EPH may be total (TH) or subtotal/supra-cervical hysterectomy (STH). STH EPH is the procedure more commonly performed (53–80%). It is faster, with less blood loss, less need for blood transfusion, less intra and post- operative complications like bladder and ureteric injury, easier for less experienced surgeons to perform of subsequent vault prolapse and retains the supports of the pelvis, thus reducing chances. The bladder and ureter are less prone to injury since they are at a safe distance from the site of dissection. It is performed for uterine rupture not extending downwards into the lower uterine segment or vaginal vault. It often is also sufficient to control bleeding in placenta previa. If, however, after clamping and ligating the uterine artery pedicles and suturing the cervical stump, bleeding continues, then the surgeon needs to proceed to total hysterectomy immediately. TH is preferred by others who aver that bleeding sometimes persists after STH from blood vessels in the cervical stump, and TH deals with such events. In the long term, TH protects against cervical neoplasia.

Considering the fact that bladder and ureteric injuries are so frequent, many surgeons precede the TH with cystoscopy and DJ stenting of the ureter to identify and protect them during the hysterectomy. These facilities may not be available in low-resource settings, in which case a careful dissection of the ureter in its pelvic course is mandated as it traverses its pelvic relations and clamping; transecting and ligating are performed under direct vision. Bleeding should be controlled before these steps are done rather than done in a morass of blood.

Emergency obstetric hysterectomy (EOH) is a challenging operation requiring senior obstetrician's intervention and participation. It is lifesaving but fraught with a number of severe complications: haemorrhage during operation from the vascular pedicles, severe thrombotic events, bladder injury, bowel injury, unintended unilateral oophorectomy, disseminated intra-vascular coagulation (DIC) and post-operative sepsis; delayed sequelae include pain syndrome; severe depression; Sheehan syndrome and fascial rupture.

The essential steps of EOH are as follows: [6].

1. Incision: Although vertical midline incision provides better exposure, if the abdomen has been opened for caesarean delivery through a transverse incision, the hysterectomy may be performed through it. If exposure needs to be improved, muscle cutting of the rectus may be done.

2. The uterus is exteriorised, and bowels packed away; bladder is protected by the abdominal retractor.

3. Round ligaments are secured separately.

4. A window is created in the broad ligament below the fallopian tube and ovarian ligament after identifying an avascular area.

5. Division and transfixion of fallopian tube and ovarian ligament

6. These upper pedicles are then secured on the opposite side.

7. Uterine arteries (UA) are skeletonised up to the by dissecting the parametrial tissue for better visualisation.

8. Firm upward traction on the cornua elevates the UA away from the ureters.

9. UA and the surrounding plexus of veins are clamped by putting clamps at the level of the LUS incision. They are cut and secured by ligatures. This is repeated on the other side.

10. Clamps are placed slightly below the level of the lower uterine segment scar/below the uterine pedicle.

11. The cervix is transected to remove the uterine corpus by circumferentially cutting around the cervix at the level of the LUS incision.

12. Cervix is oversewn with running locking sutures or multiple interlacing figures of eight sutures to ensure haemostasis and closure of the cervical canal.

13. To reduce bowel adhesions, omentum may be draped over the cervical stump.

14. All stumps are checked to ensure there is no bleeding from the cut edges or any haematoma forming on the lateral pelvic walls.

15. Intra-peritoneal drain may be considered.

16. Abdominal wall closure includes fascial and rectus sheath closure with delayed absorbable suture, fat closure with interrupted 2.0 plain catgut if thickness > 2 cm; skin may be approximated by absorbable or non-absorbable sutures or staples.

In view of the occasional necessity to perform EOH, it is imperative that all maternity OTs have instrument sets for performing hysterectomy available round-the-clock. These include abdominal retractors (Doyen. Balfour), curved and straight hysterectomy clamps (Heaney, Kochers, Zeppelin) and fine dissecting scissors (Metzenbaum). Sutures needed include polyglactin (1, 1-0,2-0), chromic catgut (1,1-0) and plain catgut (1-0) (**Figure 4**).

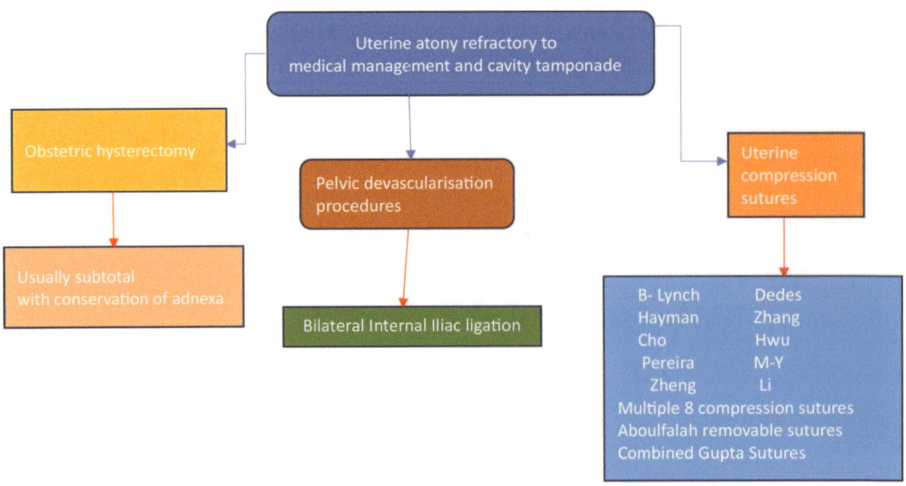

Figure 4.
Surgical procedures for refractory atonic PPH.

5.1 Damage control surgery (DCS)

The most devastating situation arises when hysterectomy also fails to control bleeding. Such a situation arises in the following:

a. When coagulopathy sets in following massive blood loss, a combination due to hypothermia (temperature less than 35°C), acidosis (pH less than 7.3) and loss of clotting factors;

b. Venous bleeding not amenable to surgical control;

c. Bleeding persists despite transfusion of large amounts of blood products (greater than 10 units packed red cells), and surgical attempts to control it have not succeeded;

d. Persistent and escalating fluid requirements not improving haemodynamic status in the setting of active non arterial bleeding;

e. Development of ventricular arrhythmias; [7] In such cases, the protocol for PPH has almost reached the end-stages, and it is extremely difficult to salvage the patient.

DCS is a linked sequence of sequences starting from aggressive support to the vital parameters followed by hysterectomy, if not previously performed, followed by packing of the abdominal cavity and finally temporal closure of the abdominal cavity. The patient is cared for post-operatively in the ICU and after 48–72 hours retaken to the operation theatre for removal of the abdominal pack, checking for dry pelvic field and final closure [8, 9].

The three cornerstones of conservative surgery include simplicity, safety and efficacy in terms of how soon and how effectively blood loss is reduced. All techniques have associated complications. Because an individual case has its own characteristics with regards to the bleeding cause and topography, surgeons should ideally have knowledge of a variety of procedures, their indications, their complications and their limitations as far as success rate is concerned.

6. Pelvic vascular procedures

Since many women who become critical due to PPH are young and would like further pregnancies, EOH, though lifesaving, would deprive them of this potential, having significant impact on their marital and familial relations. Bilateral internal iliac artery ligation (BIIAL), if successful, gives the woman the chance to preserve her fertility. It may be used in atonic PPH or even in traumatic uterine rupture PPH as an adjunct to EOH to facilitate OH and reduce reactionary haemorrhage. The first procedure was performed in 1893 by Sir Howard Kelly and was popular for many years as a less mutilating procedure for women who wished childbearing in the future.

BIIAL may be effective also in placenta previa/accreta, placental abruption and coagulopathy uterine inversion. Its success rate varies from 40 to 100%. Its limitation is that it is technically difficult, more time-taking to perform, has a long learning curve, all recommended instruments may not be available in many OTs and averts hysterectomy in only 50% cases at the expense of vital time lost.

BIIAL is effective because it reduces pelvic blood flow by almost 50% and pulse pressure by 80%, converting the pulsatile arterial circulation into a venous type stagnant blood pool facilitating clot formation to reduce bleeding.

The woman is placed in the semi-lithotomy position as it permits assessment of vaginal bleeding. The abdomen may be opened either by midline or by Pfannenstiel incision. The bowels are exteriorised and packed away. The pelvic ureter is identified at the pelvic brim. On the left side, it was sometimes necessary to incise the sigmoid mesocolon and mobilise the sigmoid colon medially in order to expose adequately the area overlying the iliac vessels. The peritoneum was incised starting from a point just proximal to the bifurcation of the common iliac artery proceeding caudally along the external iliac artery for a length of about 8 cm. The ureter was retracted with gentle blunt finger dissection, medially exposing the retroperitoneal anatomy. The fascia around the internal iliac artery is dissected carefully and completely to free the artery from its adjacent structures and to clarify the anatomical relationship of the internal iliac artery with the iliac veins. A right-angled clamp was passed beneath the internal iliac artery from lateral to medial side about 4 cm distal to its origin. As the posterior division usually branches off proximal to this, no attempt is made to locate it. Using a nonabsorbable suture (linen), the internal iliac artery was ligated singly. Pulsations of the femoral artery and dorsalis pedis were identified after tying the ligature to ensure that the correct vessel had been ligated. In cases of nontraumatic haemorrhage, once IIAL was performed, the control of haemorrhage was confirmed by improvement in vital signs as well as decrease in the amount of vaginal bleeding. If bleeding continued, hysterectomy was immediately started [10, 11].

In uterine rupture, IIAL was performed at the outset. Following this, the decision to repair the trauma or resort to hysterectomy was influenced by the extent and location of injury as well as by control of haemorrhage. In extensive vaginal lacerations, suturing was performed after IIAL so that blood loss was reduced, helping in combating shock.

The complications of BIIAL are often serious: external iliac vein injury, internal iliac vein injury, ligation of wrong structure (ureter, external/common iliac artery, external iliac artery spasm and thrombosis); rarer complications are bladder atony and necrosis of bladder mucosa or buttocks.

Pelvic devascularisation procedures got simplified when case reports appeared that procedures requiring less dissection and time could be equally effective in reducing blood loss in cases of placenta previa/accreta. The most widely used was bilateral uterine vessel ligation (O'Leary stitch). If it does succeed, then bilateral ovarian artery ligation may be done.

Tsirulnikov's triple ligation includes bilateral ligatures of the ascending branches of the uterine arteries, the utero-ovarian connections and the arteries of the round ligament (which are branches of the utero-ovarian connections [12]). Other variants are Morel's step-by-step ligation [13] and Abdrabbo sequential ligation [14].

A meta-analysis published in 2022 on 795 patients revealed the superiority of BUAL over BIIAL to control bleeding in placenta accreta spectrum patients, a condition which is rapidly becoming a common entity in obstetric emergencies given the rising rates of caesarean deliveries [15].

7. Uterine compression sutures (UCS)

These came into vogue since the late 1990s. Christopher Lynch pioneered the UCS [16]. Currently, a number of variants are being practised by obstetricians depending on their skills, preferences and familiarity [17–19]. All these effectively reduce bleeding from the placental site by the following mechanisms:

1. Direct mechanical pressure on specific bleeding uterine sites;

2. Reduces blood flow in uterine arteries.

The indications for UCS are as follows:

1. Atonic PPH during caesarean delivery not responding to uterotonics and tranexamic acid

2. Placenta praevia

3. Uterine lacerations/ rupture

4. Placenta accreta syndrome

5. Atonic PPH following vaginal delivery not responding to conservative measures including intra-uterine balloon tamponade

6. Prophylaxis of acute recurrence of uterine inversion [20, 21]

Table 2 shows the salient features of commonly performed UCS [22–28].

In order to decide the suitability of UCS for the case before proceeding with any specific procedure, the *efficacy test* should be applied to test whether the procedure will work. Manual compression of the uterus is done to see if blood loss is reduced. If positive, the surgeon goes ahead with doing the suitable procedure. If no reduction in blood loss occurs, alternative methods are resorted to immediately.

UCS classification is based on the following attributes:

1. Mode of suturing

2. Direction of suturing

3. Anatomic region of bleeding site

4. Cause of PPH

5. Whether suture transfixes uterine cavity

6. Whether sutures are removal

In addition to the procedures enumerated in Table, other procedures are also being used globally: Dedes for placenta previa/accreta during CS (circular isthmic-cervical sutures); eight compressive sutures for placenta accreta/previa; Hwu for Li 'belt-like' suture for uterine atony; placenta previa/accreta during CS (two vertical sutures on the lower segment after pushing the bladder down from in front of the suture area; Zheng (no hysterotomy, does not transfix cavity, bladder dissection not needed) [29–34].

Attribute	B-Lynch	Hayman	Cho	Pereira	Matsubara-Yano(M-Y)	ComOc-MG	Aboulfalah
Compression site	Uterine corpus	Uterine corpus	Focus region	Uterine Corpus +/− cervix	Uterine corpus	Uterine corpus	Uterine corpus
Direction of sutures	Longitu dinal	Longitu dinal	Square box-type	Around uterus long. & trans.	Criss-cross(long. & transverse	Longitudinal	longitudinal
Number of sutures	Two	Two or four	Four-five	Multiple	2/3 long. 2 transv.	Two	two
Incision on LUS	Yes	No	Yes	No	No	Yes	No
Suture material	polyglactin	polyglactin	polyglactin	polyglactin	polyglactin	polyglactin	Non absorbable
Needle type	Straight	straight	straight	Round-bodied	Straight	Round-bodied	Round-bodied
Uterine cavity obliteration	No	Yes	Yes	No	Yes	no	Yes
Removable sutures	No	No	no	No	No	No	Yes after 24–48 hrs without anaesthesia
Additional procedures	No	2 cervico-isthmic sutures	No	no	Intrauterine ballon tamponade	BUAL. ligation	+/− BUAL

BUAL: bilateral uterine artery ligation.

Table 2.
Salient characteristics of popularly performed UCS.

The efficiency of any particular compression suture depends on several factors. Studies have shown that none is superior to the others. The efficacy depends more on the proper selection for the case and how well it has performed rather than the merits of a particular technique. Overall, efficacy ranges from 60 to 100% depending on several factors like topography and cause, average being 80% [35–37]. Reduced efficacy is seen in multiparous women especially above 35 years, PPH following vaginal births and delay of more than 2–6 hours in doing the procedure.

All categories of UCS have associated complications – partial uterine ischemia, intra-cavitary synechiae, pyometra, hematometra, intestinal entrapment and uterine rupture in future pregnancies [38, 39].

During laparotomy if the bleeding is too profuse to carry on the selected procedure, some techniques are practiced to reduce blood supply to the pelvis and uterus temporarily. These include internal aortic infra-renal compression of abdominal aorta, uterine tourniquet around the lower uterine segment occluding the uterine arteries bilaterally and external compression of the uterus from fundus to LUS. These may be used for some hours in order to buy time for the patient to be transferred to a higher centre or until a specialist team arrives. The risk for uterine ischemia is significant.

8. PPH due to trauma to the reproductive tract

Trauma-causing PPH may be present at one or multiple sites in the reproductive tract. The level of trauma may range from perineum, upward into the vagina and vaginal vault, vaginal and supra-vaginal cervix, lower uterine segment and up till the upper uterine corpus and fundus with extension into the potential, highly vascular space between the layers of the broad ligament. The implication of these likely, often multiple, sites for traumatic PPH is that it is imperative that women be examined in a proper position and adequate lighting. The entire reproductive tract can then be checked for all bleeding sources. Additionally, here should be 24x7 access to operation theatre facilities where major procedures including laparotomy may be performed expeditiously where major trauma of upper reproductive tract can be managed.

Having completed a general examination of the bleeding woman and simultaneously started resuscitation to prevent systemic haemodynamic deterioration, it is mandatory to do a per abdominal examination to assess the state of uterine tonicity before proceeding to a thorough examination of the lower reproductive tract. This should not be a perfunctory exercise but should be done with the following prerequisites being fulfilled:

a. Counselling patient about the need to examine her birth canal;

b. Privacy;

c. Patient positioning, preferably in lithotomy position;

d. Adequate lighting focused on to perineum and into the vagina.

If these conditions are fulfilled in the LR, the examination may be done in the LR itself; if not, the patient is transferred to the maternity OT with informed consent to proceed to repair and manage the injury identified.

The various procedures for traumatic PPH are the following:

a. *Perineal and lower vaginal tears*: These may extend backwards to the anus or upwards up to the vaginal vault. Tears involving the lower half of vagina/perineal tears not involving the anal musculature and/or mucosa may be repaired under local anaesthesia with Vicryl 1-0. Higher order perineal tear/–s repair require transfer to MOT, regional or general anaesthesia and elaborate repair procedure by competent surgeon. The details of these techniques are beyond the scope of this chapter.

   Perineal and vaginal tears may not bleed profusely but may do so persistently. It matters to a patient whose haemoglobin is already severely lowered. Hence, they should be repaired immediately to prevent further loss, infection or any delayed complication.

b. *Cervical tears & tears of upper vagina and vaginal vault*: Every delivery room should have an adequate number of Sim's speculums and sponge-holding forceps so that bleeding sources in upper vagina and cervix may be examined adequately. If cervical tear is confirmed, its apex is visible, does not extend to the vaginal vault and does not open between the leaves of the broad ligament, the tear may be repaired in the LR itself. Vicryl 1-0 is recommended for the repair. The number of interrupted simple stitches depends on the length of the tear. It is essential to include the apex in the repair. If the apex is initially difficult to access, the repair may be commenced from below using the lower stiches for traction to pull the upper cervix into visibility till the apex is accessed and repaired.

High cervical tears extending to the vault and into the broad ligament open up the rich vascular plexus situated there, and a massive broad ligament haematoma develops rapidly, making the patient extremely pale with severely compromised vitals and hypovolemic shock [40].

9. Role of surgery in secondary PPH

Secondary PPH may sometimes be very profuse necessitating surgery if antibiotics and other medical treatments fail. Imaging of the pelvis is needed to exclude retained placenta or choriocarcinoma. Removal of placenta is often difficult since it becomes toughly adherent to the uterine wall especially in cases of placenta accreta. If evacuation attempts vaginally lead to profuse bleeding, the surgeon may have to resort to any of the surgical procedures including hysterectomy.

10. Conclusion

The two most alarming truths about PPH that explain its frontline position as a cause of maternal mortality and near-miss is that it may occur, often with alarming rapidity and severity, even in cases with no prior identifiable risk factors to red flag them; secondly, very often it occurs in low-resource settings with facilities having minimal operating infra-structure and competent manpower to follow the recommended algorithm for PPH management. Higher-order interventions like uterine artery embolization (UAE) and availability of newer pharmacological agents like recombinant activated Factor VII (rFVIIa) are present only in very few selected centres remote from the facility where the woman is bleeding post-delivery.

The above two universally accepted facts have clear management implications:

1. Since all cases who end up having PPH cannot be red-flagged in pregnancy or early labour, it is not feasible to refer them to centres where all levels of interventions are available as and when needed in the management scheme.

2. All obstetricians should be competent to decide when to go ahead with surgical interventions and be trained and conversant with various surgical procedures for PPH management.

3. Equipping maternity operation theatres with surgical instruments, anaesthetic equipment, blood transfusion facilities and consumables backed by a competent surgical and anaesthetist team and supported by an obstetric intensive care unit/ high dependency unit is a more practical and economically feasible strategy for reducing PPH mortality vis-a vis providing centres with expensive state- of-the-art setup for radiographic interventions in the form of UAE.

4. The learning curve for teaching post-graduate trainees and residents in obstetrics is shorter, less expensive and less resource-intensive compared to teaching UAE to sonography trainees.

These implications underscore the importance of including surgical techniques for controlling PPH as an essential skill to be taught to trainees in the competency-based post graduate curriculum and clinical skills checklist. This would in time translate into dramatic lowering of maternal mortality at the centres where they would be providing maternity care after completing their training.

11. Key messages

1. PPH primary or secondary often comes unannounced by any preceding warning signs or history in the antenatal or intrapartum period.

2. Risk factors for PPH need to be probed for in each patient throughout her pregnancy and labour so that a birth plan may be made regarding her place of delivery where higher-order interventions may be expeditiously available if needed.

3. All health facilities providing tertiary maternity services should have 24x7 manpower and operation theatre facilities backed by blood bank facilities and obstetric ICU/HDUs; those located in the periphery and remote regions should have a robust referral system including functioning ambulances and ambulance paramedics so that patients having PPH not responding to initial PPH care bundle may be rapidly sent to tertiary centres before they reach the irreversible shock stage.

4. Surgical management of PPH should be an integral part of the postgraduate and residency obstetric training programmes.

5. All labour rooms should have instruments to enable birth attendants to examine the lower birth canal for traumatic PPH.

6. All maternity OTs should have hysterectomy packs always ready for use.

7. Round-the-clock anaesthetist cover at tertiary maternity facilities is mandatory to provide effective care for PPH patients.

8. Clear, succinct but comprehensive information should be given to the patient and family before she is taken to the OT and an appropriate written consent taken.

9. Following the procedure, the surgeon should candidly explain the procedure and its implications regarding menstruation and reproductive functions.

Author details

Tripti Sinha
Department of Obstetrics and Gynecology, Sri Krishna Medical College, Muzaffarpur, Bihar, India

*Address all correspondence to: triptisinha0304@gmail.com

IntechOpen

© 2025 The Author(s). Licensee IntechOpen. This chapter is distributed under the terms of the Creative Commons Attribution License (http://creativecommons.org/licenses/by/4.0), which permits unrestricted use, distribution, and reproduction in any medium, provided the original work is properly cited.

References

[1] Lalonde AB, Liljestrand J, Rushwan H, Okong P. Postpartum Hemorrhage Today: Living in the Shadow of the Taj Mahal. Available from: https://www.glowm.com/pdf/PPH_2nd_edn_Chap-08.pdf

[2] World Health Organization. WHO Recommendations for the Prevention and Treatment of Postpartum Haemorrhage. Geneva: WHO; 2012. Available from: https://apps.who.int/iris/bitstream/handle/10665/75411/9789241548502_eng.pdf;jsessionid=4464904EB17B692D2D2F46B0E2BA82E3?sequence=1

[3] GBD 2015 Maternal Mortality Collaborators. Global, regional, and national levels of maternal mortality, 1990-2015: A systematic analysis for the global burden of disease study 2015. Lancet. 2016;**388**(10053):1775-1812. DOI: 10.1016/S0140-6736(16)31460-X

[4] Khan KS, Wojdyla D, Say L, et al. WHO analysis of causes of maternal death: A systematic review. Lancet. 2006;**367**(9516):1066-1074

[5] Mavrides E, Allard S, Chandraharan E, et al. Prevention and management of postpartum haemorrhage. BJOG. 2016;**124**(e106):e149

[6] Cesarean Delivery and Peripartum Hysterectomy. 26th ed. Chapter 30. William's Obstetrics. pp. 560-563

[7] Pacheco DL, Lozada MJ, Saade GR, et al. Damage-control surgery for obstetric Hemorrhage. Obstetrics and Gynecology. 2018;**132**:423-427

[8] Escobar MF, Carvajal JA, Burgos JM, et al. Damage control surgery for the Management of Major Obstetric Hemorrhage: Experience from the Fundacion Valle del Lili, Cali, Colombia. Pan-American Journal of Trauma, Critical Care and Emergency Surgery. 2017;**6**(1):1-7

[9] Waibel BH, Rotondo MM. Damage control surgery: It's evolution over the last 20 years. Revista do Colégio Brasileiro de Cirurgiões. 2012;**39**(4):314-321

[10] Joshi V, Otiv S, Majumder R, Nikam Y, Shrivastava M. Internal iliac artery ligation for arresting postpartum haemorrhage. BJOG. 2007;**114**:356-361

[11] Bellad MB. Internal iliac artery ligation (IIAL): An uterus/life-saving procedure. South Asian Federation of Obstetrics and Gynecology. 2009;**1**(2):32-33

[12] Tsirulnikov MS. Ligation of the uterine vessels during obstetrical hemorrhages. Immediate and long-term results. Journal of Gynecology Obstetrics and Human Reproduction. 1979;**8**:751-753

[13] Morel O, Malartic CJ, Muhlstein JE, et al. Pelvic arterial ligations for severe post-partum hemorrhage. Indications and techniques. Journal of Visceral Surgery. 2011;**148**:95-102

[14] Abdrabbo SA. Stepwise uterine devascularization: A novel technique for management of uncontrolled postpartum hemorrhage with preservation of the uterus. American Journal of Obstetrics and Gynecology. 1994;**171**:694-700

[15] Nabhan AE, AbdelQadir YH, Abdelghafar YA, Kashbour MO, Salem N, Abdelkhalek AN, et al. Therapeutic effect of internal iliac artery ligation and uterine artery ligation

techniques for bleeding control in placenta accreta spectrum patients: A meta-analysis of 795 patients. Frontiers in Surgery. 2022;**9**:983297. DOI: 10.3389/fsurg.2022.983297

[16] B-Lynch C, Coker A, Lawal AH, et al. The B-Lynch surgical technique for the control of massive postpartum haemorrhage: An alternative to hysterectomy? Five cases reported. British Journal of Obstetrics and Gynaecology. 1997;**104**:372-375

[17] Cho JH, Jun HS, Lee CN. Hemostatic suturing technique for uterine bleeding during cesarean delivery. Obstetrics and Gynecology. 2000;**96**(1):129-131

[18] Hayman RG, Arulkumaran S, Steer PJ. Uterine compression sutures: Surgical management of postpartum hemorrhage. Obstetrics and Gynecology. 2002;**99**(3):502-506

[19] Pereira A, Nunes F, Pedroso S, et al. Compressive uterine sutures to treat postpartum bleeding secondary to uterine atony. Obstetrics and Gynecology. 2005;**106**:569-572

[20] Matsubara S. Uterine compression suture may be useful not only for hemostasis in postpartum hemorrhage but also for prophylaxis of acute recurrence of uterine inversion. Archives of Gynecology and Obstetrics. 2010;**281**:1081-1082

[21] Matsubara S, Yano H, Ohkuchi A, et al. Uterine compression sutures for postpartum hemorrhage: An overview. Acta Obstetricia et Gynecologica Scandinavica. 2013;**92**:378-385

[22] Gupta M. COMOC-MG stitch: Modification of B-Lynch suturing technique to control atonic post-partum haemorrhage

[23] Cho JH, Jun HS, Lee CN. Hemostatic suturing technique for uterine bleeding during cesarean delivery. Obstetrics and Gynecology. 2000;**96**(1):129-131

[24] Hayman RG, Arulkumaran S, Steer PJ. Uterine compression sutures: Surgical management of postpartum hemorrhage. Obstetrics and Gynecology. 2002;**99**(3):502-506

[25] Pereira A, Nunes F, Pedroso S, et al. Compressive uterine sutures to treat postpartum bleeding secondary to uterine atony. Obstetrics and Gynecology. 2005;**106**:569-572

[26] Matsubara S, Yano H, Ohkuchi A, et al. Uterine compression sutures for postpartum hemorrhage: An overview. Acta Obstetricia et Gynecologica Scandinavica. 2013;**92**:378-385

[27] Matsubara S. A new compression suture to prevent 'uterine sandwich' from sliding off. The Australian & New Zealand Journal of Obstetrics & Gynaecology. 2012;**91**:638-639

[28] Matsubara S, Kuwata T, Baba Y, et al. A novel "uterine sandwich" for haemorrhage at cesarean section for placenta praevia. Australian and New Zealand Journal of Obstetrics and Gynaecology. 2014;**54**(3):283-286

[29] Dedes A, Ziogas V. Circular isthmic-cervical sutures can be an alternative method to control peripartum haemorraghe during caesarean section for placenta praevia accreta. Ginecologia y Obstetricia. 2008;**278**:555-557

[30] Shazly SA, Badee AY, Ali MK. The use of multiple 8 compression suturing as a novel procedure to preserve fertility in patients with placenta accreta: Case series. Australian and New Zealand Journal of Obstetrics and Gynaecology. 2012;**52**(4):395-399

[31] Hwu YM et al. Parallel vertical compression sutures: A technique to control bleeding from placenta praevia or accreta during caesarean section. Journal of Obstetrics and Gynaecology. 2005;**112**:1420-1423

[32] Li GT et al. Reflexed compression suture for the management of atonic postpartum hemorrhage with an abnormally adherent placenta. Gynecologic and Obstetric Investigation. 2015;**80**(4):228-233

[33] Zheng J et al. A new uterine compression suture for postpartum haemorrhage with atony. Journal of Obstetrics and Gynaecology. 2011;**118**:370-374

[34] Aboulfalah A et al. A new removable uterine compression by a brace suture in the management of severe postpartum hemorrhage. Frontiers in Surgery. 2014;**1**(43):1-4

[35] Doumouchtsis SK, Papageorghiou AT, Arulkumaran S. Systematic review of conservative management of postpartum hemorrhage: What to do when medical treatment fails. Obstetrical & Gynecological Survey. 2007;**62**(8):540-547

[36] Keriakos R, Chaudhuri S. Operative interventions in the management of major postpartum haemorrhage. The Obstetrician and Gynaecologist. 2012;**32**:14-25

[37] Sathe NA, Likis FE, Young JL, et al. Procedures and uterine-sparing surgeries for managing postpartum hemorrhage: A systematic review. Obstetrical & Gynecological Survey. 2016;**71**(2):99-113. DOI: 10.1097/OGX.0000000000000027

[38] Kaya B, Tuten A, Daglar K, et al. B-Lynch uterine compression sutures in the conservative surgical management of uterine atony. Archives of Gynecology and Obstetrics. 2015;**291**:1005-1014

[39] Fotopoulou C, Dudennhausen JW. Uterine compression sutures for preserving fertility in severe postpartum haemorrhage: An overview 13years after the first description. The Obstetrician and Gynaecologist. 2010;**30**(4):339-349

[40] Korde-Nayak V, Biniwale P. Broad ligament haematoma. In: Sharma A, editor. Labour Room Emergencies. Singapore: Springer; 2020. DOI: 10.1007/978-981-10-4953-8_41

Chapter 6

The Use of Mechanical Tissue Removal Devices in Hysteroscopy

Razvan Socolov, Ioana Păvăleanu, Toma Loredana, Toma Bogdan, Tudor Butureanu and Andreea Pruteanu

Abstract

The new developments in hysteroscopic surgery are increasing the advantages and decreasing the risks related to electrosurgical surgery. One of the most promising such device in the mechanical tissue removal hysteroscopic system (MTRHS), which uses simple mechanic energy to cut and aspirate intrauterine pathologies: myomas, polyps, uterine septum, retained products of conception. The advantages, when compared to the classical electrical resectoscope, are related to a minimal risk of perforation, less risk of intravasation (TURP syndrome), and faster removal. The disadvantages are pathologies that are not inside the uterine cavity, bleeding, and the need to collaborate with a pathologist because of the small fragments that are sent for examination. We critically evaluate the literature data, adding some personal experience, and conclude that the MTRHS is a promising device that could encourage young hysteroscopists to use the surgical approach.

Keywords: hysteroscopy, myomectomy, intrauterine shaver, uterine polyps, minimally invasive gynecology, hysteroscopic shaver, fertility preservation, non-electrosurgical techniques

1. The hysteroscopic tissue removal devices – Introduction

Hysteroscopic mechanical tissue removal, also known as hysteroscopic morcellation, is a procedure designed to remove submucosal uterine fibroids under direct visual guidance. This technique uses a hysteroscope, which is inserted into the uterus through the cervix, to reduce the risk of uterine trauma associated with traditional surgical methods. A key advantage over thermal ablation techniques is the elimination of the risk of thermal injury.

The hysteroscopic shaver, a specialized surgical instrument used during hysteroscopy, facilitates the precise removal of tissue from the uterine cavity. It operates with a rotating blade that cuts tissue while simultaneously suctioning the debris, enabling clear visualization and effective removal with minimal impact on healthy surrounding tissue. The shaver is used in a continuous fluid flow system to maintain visibility and minimize bleeding. This approach offers improved precision and shorter recovery times compared to traditional surgical techniques, making it ideal for removing polyps, fibroids, or other abnormal growths.

The procedure is typically performed as a day-case surgery under local, regional, or general anesthesia. A hysteroscope is inserted into the uterus through the cervix, and saline is introduced through a small channel in the hysteroscope to expand the uterine cavity. A morcellator is then passed through the hysteroscope to cut and aspirate the fibroid tissue simultaneously. The removed tissue can be collected for histological analysis, ensuring thorough evaluation and diagnosis.

Types of hysteroscopic tissue removal devices:

Presently, the double-flow bipolar resectoscope is considered the gold standard technique for performing hysteroscopic operations.

Alternative approaches to operative hysteroscopy, such as the Intrauterine Bigatti Shaver (IBS®), have been proposed to address some of the challenges associated with conventional resectoscopy. The IBS® system simultaneously removes tissue chips as they are resected, enhancing visualization during the procedure. This innovation reduces complications like fluid overload, water intoxication, uterine perforation, and the lengthy learning curve often associated with traditional techniques.

Developed in collaboration with Karl Storz GmbH & Co., the IBS® incorporates a new shaving system designed to fit through the straight operative channel of a panoramic 90° optic. This setup facilitates the performance of a wide range of major hysteroscopic procedures with improved efficiency and safety.

A study [1] included patients with various major intrauterine pathologies, such as polyps up to 6 cm and G0, G1, and G2 submucosal myomas (as per european society for gynecological endoscopy (ESGE) guidelines) up to 3 cm in diameter. Key parameters, including dilatation time, total procedural time, resection time, and fluid balance, were meticulously monitored for both patient groups. Notably, no coagulation was required, and there were no significant bleeding complications.

The study highlighted several advantages of the IBS® system. These included improved visualization due to simultaneous tissue chip removal, the absence of coagulation or cutting current requirements, the use of normal saline, and a significantly faster learning curve. Additionally, the 24 Fr diameter of the optic allowed cervical dilatation up to Hegar size 8.5, reducing the risk of cervical laceration and uterine perforation. The technique proved effective for addressing polyps and myomas up to 3 cm in diameter, offering a fast, precise, and clean approach.

However, the system faced limitations when dealing with larger, more fibrotic myomas exceeding 3 cm in diameter. To address this, two new blade designs were developed: blade number 6, with a flute-beak shape, and blade number 7, resembling shark jaws, for more aggressive cutting of fibrotic tissue.

One noteworthy case demonstrated the IBS®'s capabilities in a challenging scenario—a very large cervical G2 submucosal myoma. In this instance, the myoma, typically difficult to manage with conventional resectoscopy, was successfully removed in a two-step procedure using enhanced blade designs. This case underscores the system's potential to handle even the most complex intrauterine pathologies.

Another system developed by Medtronic is the TruClear™ dense tissue shaver.

The TruClear™ system and TruClear™ shavers are advanced medical devices designed for intrauterine use by trained gynecologists. They are specifically intended for hysteroscopic resection and removal of various intrauterine tissues, including:

- Submucous myomas
- Endometrial polyps
- Retained products of conception

Key features and description:

- Innovative cutting window: The TruClear™ dense tissue shavers feature a 10 mm open cutting window and a short distal cap, allowing precise access to intrauterine pathology in any part of the uterus.
- Oscillating blade design: The shavers operate using an oscillating-style blade that is optimized for resecting fibroids and other dense tissues.
- Variants: The TruClear™ dense tissue shaver mini and the TruClear™ dense tissue shaver plus are available for use with the corresponding TruClear™ elite hysteroscopes, offering flexibility for a range of hysteroscopic procedures.

This system combines precision and efficiency, enabling gynecologists to perform minimally invasive intrauterine tissue removal with enhanced visualization and reduced patient recovery time.

Both TruClear™ dense tissue shavers offer:

- Simultaneous tissue cutting and aspiration to reduce procedure time
- Proprietary suction control feature—suction is only activated while cutting is in progress
- 10 mm cutting window to aspirate greater volumes of tissue

The MyoSure procedure by Hologic is a straightforward and efficient method for removing intrauterine pathology. It is minimally invasive and can be conveniently performed by a doctor in an office setting. The entire procedure usually takes only 15–30 minutes, offering patients a quick and effective treatment option with minimal downtime.

Hologic offers a suite of MyoSure devices to resect and remove tissue, including a range of fibroids and polyps.

- MyoSure LITE device
- MyoSure REACH device
- MyoSure XL device
- MyoSure MANUAL device

The MyoSure procedure is a simple, efficient, in-office solution for removing intrauterine pathology. It combines precision, safety, and effectiveness, making it a preferred option for gynecological care.

Key features:

- Clear visualization: High-quality optics provide a direct, continuous view of the uterine cavity, enabling the physician to guide the procedure with confidence from start to finish.
- Tissue resection and removal: The stainless-steel blade mechanically resects unwanted tissue while the fluid management system simultaneously suctions

it out of the uterine cavity, maintaining a clear field of view throughout the procedure.

- Side-facing cutting window: Designed for optimal tissue contact, the cutting window enhances efficiency in tissue removal and reduces the risk of uterine perforation.

- Preservation of uterine function: The procedure is entirely mechanical, without the use of Radiofrequency energy. This approach preserves uterine form and function, and the collected specimens remain intact for histological analysis.

The MyoSure procedure is an effective and minimally invasive option for addressing intrauterine abnormalities while prioritizing patient safety and uterine health.

The Aquilex Fluid Control System is specifically designed to provide exceptional control and efficiency during MyoSure hysteroscopic tissue removal procedures. It works seamlessly with the MyoSure tissue removal device to enhance uterine visualization and procedural precision.

Key features:

- Optimized uterine distention: Balances steady fluid inflow with active suction to maintain optimal uterine distention, ensuring a clear and unobstructed field of view free from tissue debris.

- High-performance fluid pump: Delivers inflow rates of up to **800 ml/minutes**, enabling superior visualization of the uterine cavity during the procedure.

- Integrated dual vacuum pumps: Provides all necessary suction functions, eliminating the need for additional equipment.

- Adjustable suction control: Allows customization of suction levels for the MyoSure tissue removal device, giving precise control over the tissue removal rate to suit specific procedural needs.

The Aquilex system is an all-in-one solution that ensures efficient, safe, and effective fluid management, enhancing the overall success and ease of hysteroscopic tissue removal procedures.

Resectr by Minerva surgical:

Device description:

Resectrs are single-use, non-powered, hand-held manual surgical instruments designed for hysteroscopic procedures to dissect, resect, and remove tissue. These instruments are intended to be used as accessory tools through the working channel of an appropriately sized hysteroscope.

- Components: Resectrs consist of a non-oscillating outer cannula and an internal rotating-oscillating blade.

- Specifications: Dimensions vary based on the model number.

Intended use/indications for use:
Resectrs are intended for single-use in hysteroscopic surgical procedures for:

- Dissecting tissue
- Resecting tissue
- Removing tissue

The QuikClear RT by OriGynMED system offers a mechanical approach for the resection and removal of intrauterine tissues, eliminating the risks associated with thermal damage.

Key features:

- No thermal damage: The system employs a purely mechanical method for tissue resection, ensuring no thermal injury to the surrounding tissues.
- Immediate tissue suction: Resected tissue is suctioned and collected in a tissue trap in real-time, improving procedural efficiency and visualization.
- Safety-first design:
- No bubbles or electrical energy in the uterus, reducing the risk of air or gas embolism.
- Minimizes potential harm to the patient.
- Cutter specifications: Features a cutter with a 4 mm diameter, providing precision for intrauterine tissue removal.

System components:
The QuikClear RT system includes:

- A control unit for operational management.
- A handpiece for precise handling and tissue resection.
- A footswitch for hands-free operation and enhanced control during procedures.

This innovative system provides a safe, efficient, and precise solution for intrauterine tissue management while prioritizing patient safety.

2. Indications and clinical applications

The hysteroscopic shaver is an advanced instrument in gynecological surgery, designed to provide an efficient and minimally invasive approach to the management of intrauterine pathology. By combining mechanical cutting and tissue aspiration, it allows precise removal of abnormal tissue while preserving healthy uterine architecture. This makes it particularly valuable for treating various intrauterine conditions. Below is a detailed discussion of the key indications for its use.

Main indications for the use of the hysteroscopic shaver:

- removal of endometrial polyps, either symptomatic (causing abnormal uterine bleeding), or detected during infertility evaluation,
- resection of Type 0 or Type 1 submucosal fibroids (leiomyomas), or type 2 submucosal fibroids in selected cases, depending on size and surgeon expertise,
- management of retained products of conception after incomplete miscarriage or following failed medical or surgical evacuation procedures,
- removal of intrauterine adhesions (Asherman syndrome), to restore normal uterine anatomy and improve menstrual or reproductive outcomes,
- management of abnormal uterine bleeding (AUB) by removal of focal lesions contributing to abnormal bleeding,
- foreign body removal (most frequently displaced intrauterine devices),
- management of ectopic cesarean scar pregnancy.

Selection of cases should always consider uterine anatomy, pathology characteristics, and surgeon expertise.

2.1 Removal of endometrial polyps

Endometrial polyps are common benign pathologies of the endometrial mucosa. They can be asymptomatic but frequently manifest by abnormal AUB, including intermenstrual bleeding, menorrhagia, or postmenopausal bleeding, or as infertility, as they can obstruct the fallopian tubes and interfere with sperm transport or embryo implantation.

The hysteroscopic shaver is particularly suited for this indication as it allows for:

- precision in removal: The device can target the polyp without causing significant damage to surrounding healthy tissue,
- efficient aspiration: Simultaneous aspiration of excised tissue prevents obstruction of the surgical field and facilitates real-time visualization,
- specimen retrieval: Intact specimens are easily retrieved for histopathological evaluation, essential for ruling out malignancy, especially in postmenopausal patients.

A structured review by Yin and his team suggests that hysteroscopic removal systems have significant potential to replace conventional resectoscopy in the treatment of polyps and myomas smaller than 3 cm [2]. While their study highlights the clear advantages of hysteroscopic tissue removal systems, further clinical trials are needed to explore their potential applications in other surgical indications, such as larger myomas, uterine septa, placental remnants, and intrauterine adhesions associated with infertility treatments. An important aspect that needs to be taken into consideration is that, by minimizing thermal damage compared to traditional energy-based methods, the shaver reduces the risk of intrauterine adhesions, making it ideal for women desiring to preserve fertility [2].

In addition, intrauterine morcellation maybe associated with lower recurrence of endometrial polyps, when compared to resectoscopy [3]. To optimize the management of AUB in patients with endometrial polyps, the authors suggest that young, multiparous, or premenopausal women should be informed of their higher risk of symptom recurrence. These patients may need to explore additional treatment options for AUB following polypectomy [3].

However, the available literature data does not demonstrate the superiority of any specific method for hysteroscopic polypectomy, and no trials have been conducted specifically in infertile women. Therefore, the choice of surgical technique for hysteroscopic polypectomy should be guided by the surgeon's preference and expertise [4].

2.2 Resection of submucosal fibroids

The removal of submucosal leiomyomas is often necessary in symptomatic patients or those undergoing fertility treatments. The predominant clinical manifestations of leiomyomas in this anatomical location are menorrhagia, dysmenorrhea, and impaired fertility. The International Federation of Gynecology and Obstetrics (FIGO) classifies submucosal fibroids into:

- Type 0: Completely intracavitary.
- Type 1: Less than 50% intramural extension.
- Type 2: More than 50% intramural extension [5].

The hysteroscopic shaver has been reported to be particularly effective for Type 0 and Type 1 fibroids, mainly due to its mechanical resection, as this method avoids thermal energy, reducing the risk of uterine perforation or myometrial scarring, and also allows for controlled debulking, as the shaver allows for progressive resection of fibroid tissue, making it possible to manage fibroids of various sizes and densities. Supplementary, another advantage is the real-time visualization: continuous aspiration prevents obscuration by blood or tissue fragments, ensuring a clear view of the cavity.

In Type 2 fibroids, careful patient selection is required, and the use of preoperative uterine preparation with gonadotropin-releasing hormone (GnRH) agonists or selective progesterone receptor modulators may facilitate resection.

Regarding the actual technique and possibilities of improving it, Zhang and his colleagues performed a retrospective comparative analysis taking into account the rotational speed and the aspiration flow rate and noticed an improvement when a rotational speed of 1500 rpm with an aspiration flow rate of 500 ml/minutes was applied [6]. They showed that the hysteroscopic shaver was able to effectively enucleate myomas with a statistically significant reduction in resection time, total operative time, and fluid utilization, especially for all myomas types (0-II) smaller than 3 cm in diameter [6].

Even though the learning curve for the use of the hysteroscopic shaver is extremely short, and the surgeon's experience has little impact on the success rate of the procedure [1], myomectomy remains a complex hysteroscopic procedure and should therefore always be performed by, or under the guidance of, an experienced hysteroscopic [6].

Additionally, Ota and colleagues reported using a hysteroscopic morcellator system for the treatment of a submucosal fibroid in a patient with a history of total proctocolectomy, emphasizing the advantages of using an electrode-free device in order to minimize the risk of thermal bowel injury in patients with extensive pelvic surgery [6, 7].

2.3 Management of retained products of conception

Retained products of conception (RPOC) following miscarriage, abortion, or delivery can lead to abnormal uterine bleeding, infection, or infertility. Traditional methods such as dilatation and curettage carry a risk of excessive tissue removal, uterine perforation, adhesion formation, including Asherman syndrome, incomplete evacuation with persistence of retained intrauterine products, and curettage extending beyond the basalis layer.

In this situation, the hysteroscopic shaver offers several advantages, such as targeted tissue removal, as only retained tissue is excised, preserving the surrounding endometrium; minimized risk of adhesions in the absence of thermal injury, which is particularly useful for patients desiring future fertility; and also reduced operative time, due to the simultaneous cutting and aspirating during the procedure. This technique is particularly beneficial in managing RPOC in women with reproductive desire, those with a history of Asherman syndrome, or with a history of subfertility or a failed blind curettage [8].

2.4 Removal of intrauterine adhesions

Intrauterine adhesions result from trauma to the endometrial lining, often following infection, surgery, or uterine instrumentation. Adhesions can cause menstrual disturbances, recurrent pregnancy loss, or infertility. In this context, hysteroscopic shaver-assisted adhesiolysis is a game-changer in restoring uterine anatomy due to the precision cutting: the mechanical blade precisely separates adhesions while sparing normal endometrium. Moreover, unlike monopolar or bipolar energy devices, the shaver minimizes the risk of further endometrial injury, enhancing postoperative endometrial regeneration. The integrated aspiration system also maintains a clear operative field, even in cases with dense or vascular adhesions. As in other interventions, postoperative strategies, such as estrogen therapy or intrauterine balloon placement, can enhance recovery and prevent adhesion recurrence.

2.5 Treatment of abnormal uterine bleeding

Abnormal uterine bleeding is a frequent indication for hysteroscopy and may arise from structural abnormalities, such as polyps or fibroids, or from functional disorders. The hysteroscopic shaver is particularly effective in treating focal causes of AUB by selective tissue resection, as it can address localized lesions contributing to bleeding while preserving the surrounding endometrial architecture. Removal of suspicious lesions for histopathological analysis can aid in diagnosing malignancy or hyperplasia. The ability to perform both diagnostic and therapeutic procedures in a single session enhances patient outcomes and satisfaction.

2.6 Foreign body removal

Foreign bodies in the uterine cavity, such as displaced intrauterine devices (IUDs) or remnants of surgical materials, can cause infection, pain, or abnormal bleeding. The hysteroscopic shaver enables a safe extraction, as the device gently removes foreign materials without damaging the uterine wall and also allows concurrent tissue debridement if it is necessary.

2.7 Ectopic cesarean scar pregnancy

Liu and colleagues even reported a combined hysteroscopic shaver and resectoscope removal of a heterotopic cesarean scar pregnancy, while preserving the intrauterine pregnancy [9]. They emphasized that combining IBS with a resectoscope is an advisable method to bypass the inability of an IBS to achieve coagulation. This combination provided the advantages of a short operative time and minimal blood loss. They recommend the technique as an optimized strategy for managing heterotopic cesarean scar pregnancies in the first trimester, particularly when preservation of an intrauterine pregnancy is desired [9].

In conclusion, the hysteroscopic shaver represents a versatile and effective tool in modern gynecologic surgery. Its ability to combine mechanical resection with continuous aspiration provides significant advantages over traditional methods, particularly in terms of safety, efficiency, and precision. By minimizing thermal damage and facilitating real-time visualization, it has become a preferred option for managing intrauterine pathologies, especially in patients seeking fertility preservation. As hysteroscopic technology continues to evolve, the role of the hysteroscopic shaver is likely to expand further, offering improved outcomes for women with a wide range of gynecological conditions.

3. Limits and contraindications of hysteroscopic shaver

The hysteroscopic shaver is a highly effective tool for minimally invasive gynecological procedures, offering precision in the removal of intrauterine pathology such as polyps, fibroids, and retained products of conception. However, like any other surgical procedure, especially the minimally invasive techniques, its use is subject to certain limitations and contraindications.

Among its primary limitations is the size and location of the pathology. Large fibroids, particularly those exceeding 4–5 cm or deeply embedded into the myometrium (Type 2 or hybrid lesions), are challenging to manage effectively with the shaver [10]. Additionally, submucosal fibroids classified as FIGO type 2 or those extending into the myometrium may not be adequately removed with morcellation alone [10].

Similarly, lesions in less accessible areas, such as the cornual regions, maybe difficult to reach and remove completely. The shaver may struggle with lesions in areas such as near the uterine cornua or cervical canal [10]. The tool's efficacy also depends on optimal visualization, which can be hindered by factors such as bleeding, debris, or inadequate uterine distension [11]. Poor visualization not only compromises the procedure's success but also increases the risk of complications like uterine perforation. Additionally, the shaver is designed primarily for superficial tissue removal, making it less effective for deeply infiltrative conditions like adenomyosis.

Complex uterine anatomy also poses difficulties when handling the hysteroscopic shaver. A distorted uterine cavity due to extensive adhesions, severe endometrial atrophy, or congenital anomalies may limit the maneuverability and effectiveness of the shaver [10].

Another important limitation is the reliance on operator expertise, as the tool requires specific training for safe and effective use. The availability of equipment may also be a constraint, particularly in resource-limited settings, where the cost of disposable blades and specialized systems might pose a challenge. Despite these limitations, careful case selection and preparation can optimize outcomes.

Contraindications to the use of the hysteroscopic shaver include certain clinical scenarios that could compromise patient safety or procedural efficacy. Pregnancy is a clear contraindication due to the risk of harming the fetus or inducing pregnancy loss. Similarly, active pelvic infections, such as pelvic inflammatory disease, preclude its use, as these conditions could worsen with the procedure. Suspected malignancy presents another contraindication, as morcellation of potentially cancerous tissue may disseminate the disease. Additionally, patients with severe cervical stenosis may not tolerate the cervical dilation required for the procedure, while those with uterine perforation or a significantly thinned uterine wall face an increased risk of complications.

Medical comorbidities, such as conditions that make patients poor candidates for anesthesia or procedures with risks of fluid overload, also contraindicate the use of the shaver. Moreover, the procedure is less effective in patients with an excessively enlarged uterine cavity, which can limit proper visualization and treatment efficacy. To mitigate these risks, preoperative imaging and careful patient selection are essential. Managing fluid balance meticulously during the procedure further reduces complications, while combining the shaver with other surgical techniques may help in complex cases. Overall, while the hysteroscopic shaver is a valuable tool, understanding its limits and contraindications is crucial for ensuring safe and effective use.

Some limitations of the technique reside in the cost of the procedure. Hysteroscopic morcellation has been utilized in clinical practice for several years, but the high cost of its technology and disposable components can impose a significant financial burden on patients.

Also, there is an increased risk of bleeding, because the shaver does not coagulate blood vessels, unlike electrosurgical devices [12]. Nevertheless, this drawback may be counteracted by the combination of a hysteroscope or a resectoscope when needed [9].

To summarize, the limits of the hysteroscopic shaver are:

1. Size of lesions
2. Fibroid type
3. Visibility
4. Complex uterine anatomy
5. Limited tissue access
6. Energy-free operation
7. Operator expertise
8. Costs

Contraindications of the hysteroscopic shaver

1. Absolute contraindications:

    - Pregnancy: Hysteroscopy is contraindicated in pregnant patients due to the risk of miscarriage or uterine trauma [13],

    - Active pelvic infection: Infection increases the risk of spreading pathogens. Introducing instruments into the uterine cavity can exacerbate infections or spread them [14],

    - Malignancy suspected or confirmed uterine or cervical malignancies contraindicate morcellation due to the potential for disseminating cancerous tissue [15],

    - Severe hemorrhage or hemodynamic instability active heavy bleeding can obscure visualization, and patient instability precludes elective procedures [16].

2. Relative contraindications:

    - Severe uterine scarring: Patients with Asherman's syndrome or severe intrauterine adhesions may not be suitable due to the risk of uterine perforation or inadequate cavity expansion [12].

    - Severely distorted cavity: Significant distortion due to fibroids or congenital anomalies can make safe operation difficult [17].

    - Recent uterine surgery: Performing a shaver procedure too soon after other uterine surgeries increases the risk of complications. Prior surgical trauma or insufficient healing (e.g., after a cesarean or myomectomy) increases the risk of perforation [18].

    - Patient factors obesity or extreme uterine anteversion/retroversion can complicate access to the uterine cavity. The guidelines mention the difficulties in accessing the uterus and performing morcellation in patients with obesity or malpositioned uteri, which can lead to increased surgical time and complications [17].

3. Systemic health conditions:

- Unstable medical conditions or contraindications to anesthesia or uterine distension media, such as severe cardiac disease or pulmonary hypertension, may preclude the procedure [18].

4. Complications linked with the operative hysteroscopy using intrauterine Bigatti shaver

Hysteroscopic tissue removal systems, such as the Bigatti shaver (BS), are associated with a reduced incidence of complications, including perforation, false passage, and uterine bleeding [19]. This is attributed to their unique mechanism of action and shorter procedural duration [2]. The suction-driven, mechanically powered, rotating tubular cutting system was designed to mitigate the adverse events commonly associated with conventional resectoscopy. Hysteroscopic morcellation has been acknowledged as an efficient and safe method for the excision of intrauterine lesions such as polyps, myomas, or placental remnants, particularly in the challenging case of placenta accreta [20–22] even though cannot entire eradicate the life-threating events but the incidence appears to be less frequent when intrauterine morcellation devices are utilized, in contrast to electrocautery resection.

Types of complications:

a. Mechanical complications

Intrauterine injuries, such as uterine perforation and cervical trauma, are potential complications during hysteroscopic procedures involving the Bigatti Shaver (IBS®). Uterine perforation can occur when the instrument inadvertently punctures the uterine wall, with contributing factors including operator experience, instrument size, and the presence of uterine abnormalities such as fibroids. Cervical trauma, including lacerations or tearing, may result from improper instrument insertion or inadequate cervical dilation. To mitigate these risks, careful patient selection, the use of smaller-diameter instruments, and the employment of advanced visualization techniques are crucial [19]. Furthermore, ensuring operator proficiency through proper training and adherence to safety protocols is essential in reducing the occurrence of these complications.

A notable limitation of the bipolar hysteroscopic technique is that over 50% of uterine perforations were associated with entry, primarily due to the large diameter of conventional resectoscopes. The use of 24 Fr optical Bigatti shaver resulted in a significant reduction in entry-related complications, with an incidence of only 0.9%. In an effort to further mitigate these complications and facilitate the use of the shaver office-based settings, a novel 19 Fr optical Bigatti Shaver system was developed with better results. Using the successive described system, the need for cervical dilation in-office use is not necessary to be performed, and this initiative decreases the mechanical complications that may occur during cervical opening [19]. Jansen et al. [23] reported the incidence of uterine bleeding in 0.16% cases and highlighted that uterine perforation emerged as the most common complication, affecting approximately 0.76% of patients undergoing operative hysteroscopic procedures. Compared with conventional hysteroscopic tissue removal systems, such as resectoscopy, the complications associated with hysteroscopic morcellation, such as uterine perforation, occur in approximately 0.02% of cases, while the incidence of bleeding is reported at 0.003%.

b. Fluid-related complications

Excessive intravasation of fluid is a potential complication associated with all hysteroscopic resection techniques. The use of normal saline as a distention medium mitigates the risk of several adverse outcomes, including pulmonary and/or cerebral edema, hypo-osmolarity, and hyponatremia. These concerns are particularly significant when hyperosmolar solutions are employed. The existing literature suggests that intrauterine morcellation offers distinct advantages over traditional resectoscopy in the management of type 0, type I, or cervical submucosal myomas, according to FIGO classification [1, 21, 24]. In cases where more than 50% of the fibroid infiltrates the myometrium, such as type II myomas, increases the risk of significant intraoperative fluid absorption, as well as bleeding complications [25]. In a prospective multicenter study [23], it was established that fluid overload occurred in 0.2% of both diagnostic and operative hysteroscopic procedures performed using traditional resectoscopy techniques. The findings emphasize the importance of monitoring for potential complications during hysteroscopic procedures and the need for careful management to minimize adverse outcomes.

c. Infectious complications

Infectious complications during the use of hysteroscopic Bigatti Shaver may arise from the introduction of bacteria into the uterine cavity during the procedure. These infectious processes can manifest as endometritis, an inflammation of the uterine lining, or more severe conditions such as pelvic inflammatory disease (PID) [26]. Different factors such as retained products of conception or fibroids, which may serve as reservoirs for bacterial growth may increase the risk for uterine infection. Dilation and curettage (D&C) have historically been the standard surgical intervention for the removal of placental remnants (RPOC) but it is associated with a considerable risk of severe complications, including uterine and bowel lacerations, intrauterine adhesions (IUAs) and infectious process. Also, it is known that D&C is more frequently related with more IUAs, placental remnants, and infectious cases compared with hysteroscopy in which direct vision allows the identification and complete treatment and reduces the risk of consecutive infection [27–31].

Other factors, such as inadequate sterilization of instruments and prolonged procedure time, also contribute to raise the risk of infectious. To mitigate these risks, it is imperative to adhere to strict aseptic techniques, utilize appropriate prophylactic antibiotics, and ensure the use of fully sterilized instruments [26, 31]. Agostini et al. showed a low infectious risk after operative hysteroscopy, with no major complications during the intervention. From a total of 2116 operative interventions, they reported 1.42% rate of infections of which 0.85% cases of endometritis and 0.57% cases of urinary tract infections following hysteroscopy [32].

d. Hemorrhagic complications

Hemorrhagic complications during the use of Bigatti Shaver are relatively rare when the procedure is performed correctly. Hysteroscopic morcellators operate through mechanical energy and leverage uterine contractions to facilitate hemostasis. Hence, in instances of excessive hemorrhage, these devices do not possess electrocoagulation mechanisms or methods for cauterizing open vessels, thereby heightening the risk of substantial bleeding and fluid intravasation [25]. The inability of a BS to perform coagulation can be offset by its combination with the bipolar resectoscope [9]. In the MAUDE database, intraoperative bleeding associated with hysteroscopic morcellation was documented as 6% of the reported adverse events [25].

The principal risk factors that can contribute to hemorrhagic complications are uterine perforation, cervical laceration, endometrial or myometrial injury, placental remnants, and adhesions or fibroids [8, 33–35]. Although uterine perforation is a relatively infrequent occurrence, it can result in significant hemorrhage if large blood vessels are inadvertently affected. Cervical trauma, which may arise from improper instrument insertion or inadequate cervical dilation, can also lead to localized bleeding. Additionally, injury to the endometrial or myometrial tissue may cause substantial blood loss, particularly in areas of high vascularity. Patients with uterine abnormalities, such as fibroids or IUAs, are at a heightened risk due to the increased vascularization of these conditions. Factors that elevate the likelihood of hemorrhagic complications include the surgeon's level of experience, the duration of the procedure, and suboptimal visualization of the uterine cavity. To minimize the risk of bleeding, it is essential to implement effective hemostatic measures, such as topical agents or coagulation. Furthermore, vigilant monitoring of blood loss and fluid balance. Along with appropriate preoperative planning in high-risk cases, are critical components in managing hemorrhagic risks during hysteroscopic morcellation.

e. Anesthetic complications

Anesthetic complications associated with hysteroscopic procedures using the Bigatti Shaver are infrequent but may encompass hemodynamic disturbances such as hypotension or bradycardia, difficulties with airway management, respiratory impairments, hypersensitivity reactions to anesthetic agents, postoperative nausea and vomiting, and potential anesthetic toxicity. Furthermore, regional anesthesia may present additional risks, including nerve injury or hematoma formation. These risks can be mitigated through comprehensive preoperative evaluations, judicious selections of anesthesia techniques, and meticulous intraoperative monitoring of vital parameters, including blood pressure, oxygen saturation, and ventilation. Postoperative surveillance is essential to address complications like nausea, vomiting, or respiratory depression, ensuring optimal recovery [36].

Prevention strategies:

Critical details, such as the level of expertise of the operating physician, a clear account of how or where complications occurred, and specific management strategies for severe complications, are commonly lacking. Understanding the type of complications most likely to occur during hysteroscopic morcellation is essential for facilitating informed patient counseling and consent, while also enabling manufacturers to prioritize patient safety initiatives. The risk of complications during hysteroscopic tissue removal systems is influenced by a range of multifactorial determinants, encompassing both patient-specific characteristics and procedural variables. Optimal patient selection, thorough preoperative assessment, strict adherence to aseptic techniques, and the implementation of precise surgical techniques are critical factors in mitigating the risks associated with the procedure. Furthermore, continuous intraoperative monitoring and meticulous fluid management are essential to prevent adverse outcomes, ensuring both procedural success and patient safety.

To mitigate complications during hysteroscopic procedures utilizing the Bigatti Shaver, a multifactorial and meticulous approach is paramount. Comprehensive preoperative evaluation, including detailed imaging and patient history, is essential to identify any anatomical or pathological challenges that may complicate the procedure. Ensuring strict adherence to aseptic protocols is crucial to minimize the risk of infection, while thorough fluid management is necessary to prevent adverse events such as uterine perforation, fluid overload, or electrolyte imbalances. The surgeon must employ precise, controlled techniques during tissue removal, making use of advanced visualization technologies—such as high-definition and 3D imaging systems—that enhance real-time monitoring of the surgical site. Furthermore, continuous monitoring of uterine pressure and automated suction systems should be employed to ensure optimal tissue excision without causing undue trauma or injury. Postoperatively, vigilant observation, combined with appropriate patient education regarding potential complications, is essential for the early detection of issues such as bleeding, infection, or uterine injury. By integrating these preventive strategies, the likelihood of adverse outcomes can be significantly reduced, thereby optimizing patient safety and improving surgical efficacy.

Although life-threatening complications such as fluid overload, uterine perforation, and bleeding continue to be observed with hysteroscopic morcellation, their frequency is notably lower compared to traditional hysteroscopic resection techniques. This suggests that hysteroscopic morcellation may present a safer alternative in terms of complication rates, though ongoing vigilance and proper clinical management are imperative to mitigate potential risks.

5. Technical perspectives of development

5.1 Advancements in morcellator design

5.1.1 Improved cutting mechanism

The Bigatti Shaver employs cutting-edge technology that merges rotational blades with suction for tissue excision, providing a highly effective method for removing uterine abnormalities, such as fibroids and polyps [6, 37]. This approach significantly reduces the likelihood of thermal damage, a frequent complication encountered with conventional techniques, such as laser or electrosurgical instruments, which can inadvertently harm adjacent tissues. The blades are specifically engineered to accommodate a range of tissue consistencies, from softer endometrial layers to denser fibroids, facilitating precise and controlled tissue resection. This versatility makes the device highly adaptable, and suitable for addressing a broad spectrum of uterine conditions. Moreover, the integrated suction system efficiently evacuates excised tissue, lowering the risk of embolism and enhancing the clarity of the surgical field. These combined features make the Bigatti Shaver a highly reliable and advantageous tool in hysteroscopic procedures, offering substantial improvements over traditional resectoscopic techniques [37].

5.1.2 Compactness and maneuverability

The Bigatti Shaver's streamlined and compact design enhances its maneuverability within the uterine cavity, particularly when addressing challenging uterine fibroids located in the posterior and fundal regions, or cervical region which are often difficult to access with traditional surgical instruments [1]. The device's small diameter enables it to pass easily through the hysteroscope, maintaining the minimally invasive nature of the procedure while still providing exceptional control and precision in tissue removal. This characteristic is crucial in preserving surrounding tissue integrity, thereby reducing the risk of inadvertent damage to adjacent structures. Furthermore, the reduced size and increased flexibility of the Bigatti Shaver have led to a marked decrease in the need for more invasive surgical approaches, such as laparotomy or abdominal myomectomy. By minimizing the invasiveness of the procedure, the Bigatti Shaver contributes to improved patient outcomes, including shorter recovery times, less postoperative pain, and a reduced risk of complications typically associated with more extensive surgeries [1].

5.1.3 Multi-functionality

A notable innovation of the Bigatti Shaver is its capacity to simultaneously excise and aspirate tissue, which greatly enhances both the efficiency and safety of the procedure. This dual capability ensures the immediate removal of tissue fragments as they are cut, thereby preventing the buildup of debris within the uterine cavity that could obstruct the surgical field or elevate the risk of embolism. The continuous suction not only aids in the prompt evacuation of tissue but also helps to control bleeding by maintaining a clear surgical site. This constant suction improves visibility, allowing the surgeon to operate with greater precision and accuracy. The combined action of cutting and aspiration reduces the likelihood of complications, offering a more effective and safer alternative to conventional methods that lack such integrated functions [2, 6, 37].

5.1.4 Material and durability

The Bigatti Shaver is fabricated from premium materials designed to provide long-lasting durability while preserving its sharpness over extended use. This is essential for ensuring reliable performance during protracted surgical procedures. The use of high-grade stainless steel and other corrosion-resistant materials contributes to the instrument's longevity, ensuring that it retains its cutting-edge across multiple procedures, thus maintaining optimal functionality throughout its lifespan [2, 37].

5.2 Visualization technology in hysteroscopy

5.2.1 High-definition and 3D visualization

The continuous advancement of high-definition hysteroscopic technology has significantly enhanced the visual clarity of the uterine cavity, enabling surgeons to observe intricate details with greater precision. This enhancement in visualization facilitates more accurate identification of fibroids, polyps, and other uterine abnormalities. Recent innovations, such as three-dimensional (3D) imaging, further augment this capability by providing a comprehensive view of the uterine structure in three dimensions. This advancement improves the precision of tissue resection, particularly in cases involving larger fibroids or when operating in complex anatomical regions, thereby enhancing the overall efficacy and safety of the procedure [2, 35].

5.2.2 Miniaturization of the hysteroscope

Recent advancements have led to the development of more compact and sophisticated hysteroscopes, broadening the patient population eligible for hysteroscopic morcellation. These miniaturized devices enhance patient comfort and minimize the likelihood of uterine injury, while still providing superior imaging quality. Additionally, the reduction in instrument size enhances the flexibility and maneuverability of the tools, allowing surgeons to navigate the uterine cavity with greater ease and effectively access fibroids located in the most challenging areas [19].

5.2.3 Integration of robotics and automation

5.2.3.1 Robot-assisted hysteroscopy

Recent technological advancements have facilitated the integration of robotic-assisted systems into hysteroscopic surgery, offering significant improvements in both precision and control during procedures. These robotic platforms enable enhanced stability and accuracy when operating the morcellator, which is particularly advantageous in complex or challenging clinical scenarios. The utilization of robotic systems helps mitigate the effects of tremor and surgeon fatigue, which are common drawbacks in traditional manual operations, thereby contributing to improved surgical outcomes for both patients and practitioners. Furthermore, robotic systems are typically equipped with advanced visualization technologies, offering superior imaging clarity, and ergonomic features that optimize the surgeon's posture and reduce physical strain. The ability to perform highly precise movements with minimal invasiveness ensures greater safety and efficiency in uterine surgeries, making robotic assistance a valuable tool in modern gynecological procedures [38, 39].

5.2.3.2 Automation in morcellation

Recent advancements in morcellator technology have led to the incorporation of automated features, such as automatic blade adjustments that respond to tissue density or feedback from the excised material. These innovations contribute to optimizing cutting speed, reducing the likelihood of tissue fragmentation, and enhancing the overall efficiency of the procedure. Additionally, automation plays a pivotal role in monitoring the surgical process by providing real-time data on key parameters, including the volume of tissue removed, the extent of bleeding, and the overall success of the operation. This integration of real-time feedback not only ensures more precise control during the procedure but also contributes to better patient outcomes by enabling dynamic adjustments throughout the course of the surgery [2, 35, 37].

5.3 Energy-based technology

5.3.1 Combination with electrosurgery

While the Bigatti Shaver predominantly utilizes a mechanical cutting mechanism, ongoing innovations are focused on integrating morcellation with other energy-based modalities, such as electrosurgery or laser technology. These complementary technologies assist in controlling hemorrhage and enhancing precision during tissue excision. The development of hybrid morcellators has further advanced this approach, allowing the surgeon to seamlessly alternate between various techniques, such as mechanical cutting and electrosurgical coagulation. This flexibility enables the practitioner to tailor the surgical method according to the tissue characteristics or the specific pathological condition being addressed, ultimately improving procedural outcomes and patient safety [40].

5.3.2 Minimizing heat generation

A critical technical consideration in the advancement of contemporary morcellators is the reduction of thermal injury to adjacent tissues. The generation of excessive heat during the morcellation process poses significant risks, including uterine burns and damage to the endometrial lining, which can result in adverse clinical outcomes. Consequently, recent iterations of morcellators are meticulously designed to operate with minimal heat production, thereby safeguarding surrounding tissues from inadvertent thermal harm. This focus on temperature control not only enhances the safety profile of the device but also contributes to improved procedural precision and patient outcomes [37, 41].

5.4 Safety features and risk mitigation

5.4.1 Pressure-controlled systems

Modern hysteroscopic systems, including the Bigatti Shaver, often feature pressure-controlled suction mechanisms to avoid excessive uterine distension, which could lead to complications like uterine perforation or fluid overload (especially with the use of distension media). Some morcellators are now designed with automated pressure sensors that adjust the suction force in real-time, ensuring that the tissue is removed effectively without compromising patient safety [37].

5.5 Patient-specific customization

5.5.1 Personalized instrumentation

The technical development of hysteroscopic morcellation tools now allows for customized settings tailored to each patient's specific anatomical and medical condition. For example, the morcellator's cutting speed, suction power, and blade size can be adjusted based on the size and location of the fibroid or polyp.

Advanced systems can also incorporate patient-specific data (like uterine size and fibroid location) into the procedure planning, helping optimize the surgical approach and improve the likelihood of a successful outcome [37].

5.6 Postoperative monitoring and imaging

5.6.1 Real-time feedback

Some newer systems provide real-time feedback to the surgeon regarding the effectiveness of the tissue removal, including parameters such as tissue consistency, volume, and any complications like bleeding or incomplete removal. Postoperative imaging, such as ultrasound or MRI, is being increasingly integrated into hysteroscopic procedures to provide better postoperative assessment, enabling better decision-making and follow-up care [42].

5.7 Future directions

The future of hysteroscopic morcellation with the Bigatti Shaver and similar technologies lies in increased automation, improved safety features, advanced imaging systems, and smarter integration of robotic and AI systems. As the technology continues to evolve, we can expect even more precise, safe, and patient-friendly surgical techniques with reduced complication rates and faster recovery times. These technical developments hold the promise of transforming the field of minimally invasive gynecological surgery, making it more accessible and effective for patients worldwide [38, 39].

6. Uterine mechanical tissue removal devices vs. hysteroscopic resectoscope: Understanding the differences in treating uterine pathology

Advances in minimally invasive gynecology have transformed the treatment of intrauterine pathologies, such as submucosal fibroids, endometrial polyps, and retained products of conception. Historically, the hysteroscopic resectoscope (HR) was the gold standard for these procedures. However, the development of uterine mechanical tissue removal devices (UMTRDs) has introduced a modern alternative, offering distinct advantages and limitations. Understanding the differences between these techniques is crucial for tailoring treatment to each patient's unique needs.

Hysteroscopic resectoscope has been a reference in gynecological intrauterine surgery for decades. This instrument uses a combination of visualization, cutting, and coagulation capabilities to remove intrauterine pathology. Powered by either monopolar or bipolar energy, it requires continuous fluid distension of the uterine cavity, allowing the surgeon to view and excise abnormal tissue with precision.

In contrast, uterine mechanical tissue removal devices represent a newer generation of technology. Devices such as IBS™, MyoSure™, and TruClear™ employ mechanical cutting blades housed within a protective sheath, integrated with a suction system. This design facilitates simultaneous tissue cutting and evacuation without the use of electrosurgery. The UMTRDs are particularly valued for their simplicity and efficiency, offering a potentially safer and faster alternative to the resectoscope for certain pathologies.

6.1 How they differ: Key features

At first glance, the hysteroscopic resectoscope and UMTRDs may appear similar because they both rely on hysteroscopic visualization. However, the nuances of their mechanisms set them apart. The resectoscope employs electrical energy for cutting and coagulation, making it suitable for vascular lesions where bleeding control is essential. The moves required by the surgeon are related to "cut under vision" procedures, so the safety of any intervention needs good visualization of both the lesion, the operating tip of the resectoscope, and the uterine wall.

On the other hand, UMTRDs use mechanical blades to excise tissue, which is then aspirated during the procedure. The procedure is more related to appropriate contact between the blades and the lesion, therefore the need for panoramic visualization or the permanent observation of the operating instrument in its relation to the uterine wall is less important. This could provide a certain safety feeling to the surgeon, even from the early learning curve.

The need for electrosurgery with the resectoscope introduces certain risks, such as thermal injury to adjacent tissue. UMTRDs, which operate without electricity, mitigate this risk, making them particularly appealing in cases where preservation of the uterine environment is critical, such as for women planning future pregnancies.

6.2 Advantages of the hysteroscopic resectoscope

One of the primary strengths of the hysteroscopic resectoscope is its versatility. It excels in treating complex and large intrauterine pathologies, including intracavitary or submucosal fibroids larger than 3 cm. Surgeons trained in its use can achieve excellent results even in challenging cases.

Additionally, the resectoscope's ability to simultaneously cut and coagulate tissue helps minimize bleeding during the procedure, making it a reliable tool for managing vascularized lesions. It is also cost-effective for high-volume practices since the instrument is reusable and has long been a staple in gynecology.

However, these benefits come with trade-offs. Mastering the resectoscope requires a significant learning curve, and complications such as uterine perforation or thermal injury remain potential risks. Moreover, the use of fluid for uterine distension necessitates careful monitoring to avoid complications like fluid overload or hyponatremia, particularly when monopolar systems require nonionic media.

UMTRDs have gained popularity due to their simplicity and safety. Their mechanical cutting mechanism eliminates the need for electrosurgery, thereby reducing risks associated with thermal damage. This makes them particularly suitable for less experienced operators or for outpatient settings where simpler procedures are preferred.

The efficiency of UMTRDs is another major advantage. Unlike the resectoscope, which often requires manual retrieval of excised tissue, UMTRDs incorporate a suction system that continuously removes tissue during the procedure. This streamlining reduces operative time, which can be beneficial for both the patient and the surgical team.

Patient comfort is another noteworthy aspect. Studies have shown that procedures using UMTRDs are often better tolerated under local anesthesia or conscious sedation, potentially eliminating the need for general anesthesia in many cases [21]. This can translate to shorter recovery times and lower overall healthcare costs.

Despite these benefits, UMTRDs are not without limitations. Their efficacy diminishes when addressing larger or more complex lesions. For instance, submucosal fibroids exceeding 3 cm may be challenging to remove completely with UMTRDs. Additionally, the proprietary nature of these devices, often involving single-use components, can make them more expensive than resectoscopes in the long run.

6.3 Clinical outcomes: How do they compare?

In terms of efficacy, both UMTRDs and the hysteroscopic resectoscope demonstrate excellent outcomes for smaller fibroids and polyps. A meta-analysis comparing the two methods revealed comparable rates of symptom resolution, with UMTRDs offering shorter procedure times [43]. However, for larger lesions or those requiring extensive removal, the resectoscope continues to outperform UMTRDs in achieving complete resection.

Regarding the operative data parameters, a large meta-analysis done by Ren [44] studied the results of six RCTs comparing hysteroscopic morcellation and conventional resectoscopy. According to this article, there are no significant differences between the two procedures in terms of success rate and fluid deficit. The operation time was a bit shorter in the morcellation group (2.81 minutes average for the surgical time, and 3.43 minutes for the whole procedure). It is worth mentioning that all RCTs included the same brand morcellator, and no bias was determined in the analysis.

The completion of the procedure is another issue that is discussed as a comparison between the two procedures. As shown by Sivas et al. [45] in the case of UMTRD or resectoscope use for polypectomy, a pathological evaluation of the remaining bed of the polyp (by curettage) showed that 7 out of 35 patients still had polypoid tissue in the curettage specimen, although completion of the procedure was certified by visual inspection. Despite the other advantages mentioned by the authors of this RCT, like less blood loss and shorter intervention time, an increased fluid deficit (500 ml vs. 300 ml), and this risk of leaving the bed of the lesion was mentioned.

Safety profiles also differ. While both techniques have low complication rates overall, UMTRDs boast a better safety profile for straightforward cases due to the elimination of electrosurgical risks. On the other hand, some lesions, like fibrotic leiomyomas, especially type 2, may prove too difficult for the blade of the morcellator to be efficient, and the surgeon is required to switch to a resectoscope, as shown by the article of van Wessel et al. [34]. Therefore, the surgeon should be familiar with both techniques in cases of large, calcified fibroids.

Patient recovery and satisfaction further highlight the strengths of UMTRDs. Many patients experience shorter recovery times and less postoperative discomfort after procedures performed with mechanical tissue removal devices, likely due to the minimally invasive nature of the technology [46]. However, this advantage may be less pronounced in cases requiring more extensive surgical intervention, where the versatility of the resectoscope becomes essential. The use of a miniresectoscope or of new smaller-diameter hysteroscopic morcellators is an important step toward in-office myomectomies, associated with higher patient satisfaction [47].

6.4 Choosing the right tool

Selecting between the hysteroscopic resectoscope and UMTRDs is often a matter of balancing the complexity of the pathology with the surgeon's expertise and the patient's needs. For simpler cases, such as the removal of small endometrial polyps or retained products of conception, UMTRDs offer a safer and faster option with less risk of complications. For larger, vascular, or more complex lesions, the hysteroscopic resectoscope remains the tool of choice.

The surgeon's skill level and familiarity with the instruments also play a significant role. While the resectoscope demands extensive training and practice, UMTRDs are more user-friendly, making them accessible to a broader range of practitioners.

6.5 Financial aspects

The purchase of UMTRD equipment is an important financial decision. Besides the different advantages and limitations discussed throughout this chapter, the price of equipment which is added to the hysteroscopy line (which often includes also resectoscope) is an issue that medical administrations could raise.

In the retrospective analysis done by Jamdade et al. [48] over 58 outpatient hysteroscopic morcellation procedures in 1 year, the financial saving in average was 1117 GBP per case. This is due, of course, to the outpatient settings, but also to recovery and perioperative management.

7. Conclusion

Hysteroscopic morcellation has been recently introduced in many gynecological units. It has several advantages but also limits that the specialists should be aware of when compared to resectoscopes. In more difficult cases, the combination of both methods is required either because of the size or location of the pathology or by solving some hemorrhagic lesions.

Both the hysteroscopic resectoscope and uterine mechanical tissue removal devices have revolutionized the treatment of intrauterine pathology. By understanding the strengths and limitations of each method, gynecologists can make informed decisions that optimize patient outcomes.

Author details

Razvan Socolov[1,2], Ioana Păvăleanu[1,2]*, Toma Loredana[1,2], Toma Bogdan[1], Tudor Butureanu[1,2] and Andreea Pruteanu[1,2]

1 Department of Mother and Child Medicine, University of Medicine and Pharmacy Grigore T Popa, Iasi, Romania

2 Hospital of Obstetrics and Gynecology Elena Doamna, Iasi, Romania

*Address all correspondence to: ioana_pavaleanu@yahoo.com

IntechOpen

© 2025 The Author(s). Licensee IntechOpen. This chapter is distributed under the terms of the Creative Commons Attribution License (http://creativecommons.org/licenses/by/4.0), which permits unrestricted use, distribution, and reproduction in any medium, provided the original work is properly cited.

References

[1] Bigatti G, Ferrario C, Rosales M, et al. A 4-cm G2 cervical submucosal myoma removed with the IBS® integrated Bigatti shaver. Gynecological Surgery. 2012;**9**(4):453-456

[2] Yin X, Cheng J, Ansari SH, Campo R, Di W, Li W, et al. Hysteroscopic tissue removal systems for the treatment of intrauterine pathology: A systematic review and meta-analysis. Facts, Views & Vision in ObGyn. 2018;**10**(4):207-213

[3] AlHilli MM, Nixon KE, Hopkins MR, Weaver AL, Laughlin-Tommaso SK, Famuyide AO. Long-term outcomes after intrauterine morcellation vs hysteroscopic resection of endometrial polyps. Journal of Minimally Invasive Gynecology. 2013;**20**(2):215-221. DOI: 10.1016/j.jmig.2012.10.013. Epub 2013 Jan 5

[4] Tanos V, Berry KE, Seikkula J, Abi Raad E, Stavroulis A, Sleiman Z, et al. The management of polyps in female reproductive organs. International Journal of Surgery. 2017;**43**:7-16. DOI: 10.1016/j.ijsu.2017.05.012. Epub 2017 May 5

[5] Munro MG, Critchley HO, Broder MS, Fraser IS, FIGO Working Group on Menstrual Disorders. FIGO classification system (PALM-COEIN) for causes of abnormal uterine bleeding in nongravid women of reproductive age. International Journal of Gynaecology and Obstetrics. 2011;**113**(1):3-13. DOI: 10.1016/j.ijgo.2010.11.011. Epub 2011 Feb 22

[6] Zhang S, Di W, Wang Y, Shi J, Yin X, Zhang Y, et al. Hysteroscopic myomectomy with the IBS® intrauterine Bigatti shaver: A retrospective comparative analysis of the impact of rotational speed and aspiration flow rate. Facts, Views & Vision in ObGyn. 2023;**15**(1):53-59. DOI: 10.52054/FVVO.15.1.063

[7] Ota K, Takahashi T, Kamo N, Endo Y, Furukawa S, Soeda S. Successful management of a submucosal fibroid using a hysteroscopic morcellator system in a patient with a history of total proctocolectomy: A case report. The Journal of Obstetrics and Gynaecology Research. 2020;**46**(11):2450-2453. DOI: 10.1111/jog.14481. Epub 2020 Sep 10

[8] Sutherland NSV, Rajesh H. The intrauterine Bigatti shaver system: An alternative option for focal retained products of conception. Case Reports in Obstetrics and Gynecology. 2018;**2018**:1536801. DOI: 10.1155/2018/1536801

[9] Liu W, Yue Y, Hou X, Han H, Wang W, Lin X. Combined hysteroscopic Bigatti shaver (IBS) and resectoscope removal of a heterotopic cesarean scar pregnancy in the first trimester. Fertility and Sterility. 2024;**122**(3):546-548. DOI: 10.1016/j.fertnstert.2024.04.024. Epub 2024 Apr 25

[10] Di Spiezio SA, Bettocchi S, Spinelli M, Guida M, Nappi L, Angioni S, et al. Review of new office-based hysteroscopic procedures 2003-2009. Journal of Minimally Invasive Gynecology. 2010;**17**(4):436-448. DOI: 10.1016/j.jmig.2010.03.014

[11] Lasmar RB, Barrozo PR, Dias R, Oliveira MA. Submucous myomas: A new presurgical classification to evaluate the viability of hysteroscopic surgical treatment–Preliminary report. Journal of Minimally Invasive Gynecology. 2005;**12**(4):308-311. DOI: 10.1016/j.jmig.2005.05.014

[12] Campo R, Santangelo F, Gordts S, et al. Outpatient hysteroscopy. Facts, Views & Vision in Obgyn. 2018;**10**(3):115-122

[13] Shah DK et al. Hysteroscopy and pregnancy: Risks and recommendations. Fertility and Sterility. 2014;**102**(5):1248-1253

[14] Bosteels J, van Wessel S, Weyers S, Broekmans FJ, D'Hooghe TM, Bongers MY, et al. Hysteroscopy for treating subfertility associated with suspected major uterine cavity abnormalities. Cochrane Database of Systematic Reviews. 2018;**12**(12):CD009461. DOI: 10.1002/14651858.CD009461.pub4

[15] Parker WH. Indications for morcellation in gynecologic surgery. Current Opinion in Obstetrics and Gynecology. Feb 2018;**30**(1):75-80. DOI: 10.1097/GCO.0000000000000427

[16] Yang LC, Chaudhari A. ACOG Practice Bulletin Number 800 Hemorrhage and Surgical Management in Gynecologic Procedures. Mar 2020;**135**(3):138-148

[17] Loddo A, Djokovic D, Drizi A, De Vree BP, Sedrati A, van Herendael BJ. Hysteroscopic myomectomy: The guidelines of the International Society for Gynecologic Endoscopy (ISGE). European Journal of Obstetrics & Gynecology and Reproductive Biology. 2022;**268**:121-128. ISSN 0301-2115. DOI: 10.1016/j.ejogrb.2021.11.434

[18] American College of Obstetricians and Gynecologists (ACOG). Practice bulletin No. 154: Uterine surgery and its impact on future fertility and reproductive outcomes. Obstetrics & Gynecology. 2016;**127**(3):636-642

[19] Bigatti G, Ansari SH, Di W. The 19 Fr. Intrauterine Bigatti shaver (IBS®): A clinical and technical update. Facts, Views & Vision in ObGyn. 2018;**10**(3):161-164

[20] Emanuel MH et al. The intra uterine morcellator: A new hysteroscopic operating technique to remove intrauterine polyps and myomas. Journal of Minimally Invasive Gynecology. 2005;**12**(1):62-66

[21] Hamerlynck TWO, Dietz V, Schoot BC. Clinical implementation of the hysteroscopic morcellator for removal of intrauterine myomas and polyps. A retrospective descriptive study. Gynecological Surgery. 2011;**8**:193-196

[22] Shi J, Zhang Y, Zhang S, Yin X, An D, Zhang J, et al. Intrauterine Bigatti shaver (IBS ®) successful placental remnants removal, after caesarean section for a cervical pregnancy with placenta accreta. Facts, Views & Vision in ObGyn. 2022;**14**(1):95-98. DOI: 10.52054/FVVO.14.1.010

[23] Jansen FW, Vredevoogd CB, van Ulzen K, Hermans J, Trimbos JB, Trimbos-Kemper TC. Complications of hysteroscopy: A prospective, multicenter study. Obstetrics and Gynecology. 2000;**96**(2):266-270. DOI: 10.1016/s0029-7844(00)00865-6

[24] Knipe H, Hapugoda S, Elfeky M, et al. FIGO Classification System for Uterine Leiomyoma. Reference Article. Radiopaedia.org. DOI: 10.53347/rID-156167 [Accessed: December 24, 2024]

[25] Haber K, Hawkins E, Levie M, Chudnoff S. Hysteroscopic morcellation: Review of the manufacturer and user facility device experience (MAUDE) database. Journal of Minimally Invasive Gynecology. 2015;**22**(1):110-114. DOI: 10.1016/j.jmig.2014.08.008. Epub 2014 Aug 14

[26] Cicinelli E, Cicinelli R, Vitagliamo A. Chapter 18—Infective complications: Risk, diagnosis, and treatment. In: Manchanda R, Laganà AS, editors. Complications of Hysteroscopy. Elsevier; 2024. pp. 257-267. ISBN:9780443216169

[27] Hooker AB, Aydin H, Brölmann HA, Huirne JA. Long-term complications and reproductive outcome after the management of retained products of conception: A systematic review. Fertility and Sterility. 2016;**105**(1):156-64.e1-2. DOI: 10.1016/j.fertnstert.2015.09.021. Epub 2015 Oct 9

[28] Pather S, Ford M, Reid R, Sykes P. Postpartum curettage: An audit of 200 cases. The Australian & New Zealand Journal of Obstetrics & Gynaecology. 2005;**45**(5):368-371. DOI: 10.1111/j.1479-828X.2005.00445.x

[29] Golan A, Dishi M, Shalev A, Keidar R, Ginath S, Sagiv R. Operative hysteroscopy to remove retained products of conception: Novel treatment of an old problem. Journal of Minimally Invasive Gynecology. 2011;**18**(1):100-103. DOI: 10.1016/j.jmig.2010.09.001

[30] Ansari SH, Bigatti G, Aghssa MM. Operative hysteroscopy with the Bigatti shaver (IBS®) for the removal of placental remnants. Facts, Views & Vision in ObGyn. 2018;**10**(3):153-159

[31] Aas-Eng MK, Langebrekke A, Hudelist G. Complications in operative hysteroscopy—Is prevention possible? Acta Obstetricia et Gynecologica Scandinavica. 2017;**96**(12):1399-1403. DOI: 10.1111/aogs.13209. Epub 2017 Sep 27

[32] Agostini A, Cravello L, Shojai R, Ronda I, Roger V, Blanc B. Postoperative infection and surgical hysteroscopy. Fertility and Sterility. 2002;**77**(4):766-768. DOI: 10.1016/s0015-0282(01)03252-6

[33] Cooper J, Brady RM. Late complications of operative hysteroscopy. Obstetrics and Gynecology Clinics of North America. 2000;**27**:367-374. DOI: 10.1016/S0889-8545(00)80027-3

[34] van Wessel S, van Vliet HAAM, Schoot BC, Weyers S, Hamerlynck TWO. Hysteroscopic morcellation versus bipolar resection for removal of type 0 and 1 submucous myomas: A randomized trial. European Journal of Obstetrics, Gynecology, and Reproductive Biology. 2021;**259**:32-37. DOI: 10.1016/j.ejogrb.2021.01.050. Epub 2021 Jan 29

[35] Noventa M, Ancona E, Quaranta M, Vitagliano A, Cosmi E, D'Antona D, et al. Intrauterine morcellator devices: The icon of hysteroscopic future or merely a marketing image? A systematic review regarding safety, efficacy, advantages, and contraindications. Reproductive Sciences. 2015;**22**(10):1289-1296. DOI: 10.1177/1933719115578929. Epub 2015 Apr 14

[36] Elahmedawy H, Snook NJ. Complications of operative hysteroscopy: An anaesthetist's perspective. BJA Education. 2021;**21**(7):240-242. DOI: 10.1016/j.bjae.2021.03.001. Epub 2021 May 6

[37] Franchini M, Ceci O, Casadi P, Carugno J, Giarrè G, Gubbini G, et al. Mechanical hysteroscopic tissue removal or hysteroscopic morcellator: Understanding the past to predict the future. A narrative review. Facts, Views & Vision in ObGyn. 2021;**13**(3):193-201

[38] Harvey L, Hendrick R, Dillon N, Blum E, Branscombe L, Webster S, et al. A novel robotic endoscopic device used for operative hysteroscopy. Journal of Minimally Invasive Gynecology. 2020;**27**(7):1631-1635

[39] Isaacson K. Robotic hysteroscopy: Sounds crazy, No? Journal of

Minimally Invasive Gynecology. 2020;**27**(7):1441-1442

[40] Iavazzo C, Fotiou A, Kokkali K, Gkegkes ID. Transvaginal morcellation: Tips and tricks and the role of "Iavazzo score". Archives of Gynecology and Obstetrics. 2024;**310**(4):2293-2294

[41] Vitale SG, Haimovich S, Riemma G, Ludwin A, Zizolfi B, De Angelis MC, et al. Innovations in hysteroscopic surgery: Expanding the meaning of "in-office". Minimally Invasive Therapy & Allied Technologies. 2021;**30**(3):125-132

[42] Wagenaar LP, van Vliet HA, Radder CM, Peters LW, Weyers S, Schoot BC, et al. Operative hysteroscopy versus ultrasound-guided electric vacuum aspiration for removal of retained products of conception: A prospective cohort study. European Journal of Obstetrics & Gynecology and Reproductive Biology: X. 2023;**20**:100230

[43] Smith AJ et al. Comparative outcomes of hysteroscopic resectoscope and mechanical tissue removal devices: A meta-analysis. Journal of Minimally Invasive Gynecology. 2018;**25**(3):1-10

[44] Ren F, Huang G, Wang X, Li X, Cai J. Comparison of hysteroscopic morcellation versus resectoscopy in treatment of patients with endometrial lesions: A meta-analysis. Medical Science Monitor. 2022;**28**

[45] Sivas MC, Ohanoglu Cetinel K, Arslan HS. Evaluation of whether there is residual polyp tissue after hysteroscopic morcellation at Cam and Sakura City Hospital: A retrospective cohort study. BMC Women's Health. 2024;**24**(1):133

[46] Vilos GA et al. Advances in the treatment of submucosal fibroids: Role of mechanical tissue removal devices. Fertility and Sterility. 2021;**116**(2):312-320

[47] Valero I, García-Jiménez R, Florez N, Weber-Fernandez AM, Oña López MR, Lara MD. Mini-resectoscope vs morcellator for in-office hysteroscopic myomectomy: Evaluation of results and patient satisfaction. European Journal of Obstetrics, Gynecology, and Reproductive Biology. 2022;**270**:95-99

[48] Jamdade K, Opokuansah P, Kalkur S. Evaluation of efficacy and cost-effectiveness of outpatient resection of endometrial pathologies in a university hospital in the UK. Journal of Mid-Life Health. 2024;**15**:182-187

Section 4

Postsurgical Management

Chapter 7

Postoperative Care

Visar Disha

Abstract

The topic of "Postoperative Care" focuses on the essential medical practices and protocols followed after a surgical procedure to ensure patient recovery and minimize complications. This chapter will explore various aspects of postoperative care, including pain management, wound care, monitoring vital signs, and preventing infections. It will also address the psychological aspects of recovery, patient education, and rehabilitation strategies to promote healing and improve long-term outcomes. The scope of the chapter covers both immediate postoperative interventions and extended care practices, highlighting their importance in reducing morbidity and mortality. Furthermore, it will discuss the role of healthcare providers in ensuring successful patient recovery post-surgery.

Keywords: postoperative care, pain management, wound care, patient recovery, rehabilitation strategies

1. Introduction

Postoperative care is the management and monitoring of patients after surgery to ensure a smooth recovery and prevent complications. It is a multidisciplinary process that involves a wide range of healthcare professionals, including surgeons, anesthesiologists, nurses, and physiotherapists. The goals of postoperative care include pain management, early detection of complications, ensuring proper wound healing, and helping patients return to normal activities. Inadequate postoperative care can lead to increased morbidity, mortality, and healthcare costs [1]. This chapter aims to provide an in-depth exploration of postoperative care, including different phases, strategies for pain management, wound care, infection prevention, and the psychological and educational aspects of care. The chapter also highlights the importance of tailored care plans based on the patient's individual needs and type of surgery performed.

2. Phases of postoperative care

Postoperative care can be divided into three main phases: The immediate, intermediate, and extended phases. Each phase requires specific interventions to ensure a smooth recovery.

2.1 Immediate postoperative phase

The immediate postoperative phase refers to the first few hours after surgery, usually spent in the post-anesthesia care unit (PACU). During this phase, the patient's condition is closely monitored, and interventions focus on stabilizing vital signs, managing pain, and preventing early complications.

- Monitoring vital signs: Close monitoring of vital signs is crucial in this phase. A sudden drop in blood pressure, rapid heart rate, or low oxygen saturation can indicate complications such as hemorrhage, hypovolemia, or respiratory distress [2].

- Airway management and Respiratory Support: In the immediate phase, the patient may still be under the effects of anesthesia, making airway management essential. Some patients may require supplemental oxygen or mechanical ventilation, especially after major surgeries or procedures involving the chest or abdomen [3].

- Pain control: Managing pain is critical to preventing postoperative complications such as cardiovascular stress or impaired breathing. A multimodal approach, including opioid and non-opioid analgesics, is often used to manage pain effectively [4].

2.2 Intermediate postoperative phase

This phase typically begins once the patient is stable and able to move out of the PACU, continuing through the first few days post-surgery. The focus shifts toward early mobilization, infection prevention, and supporting the body's healing processes.

- Wound management: Regular dressing changes and inspections for signs of infection or dehiscence (wound reopening) are crucial. Wounds healing by primary or secondary intention should be monitored closely, and healthcare providers must ensure sterile techniques to prevent infections [5].

- Early mobilization: Immobility increases the risk of complications such as deep vein thrombosis (DVT), pulmonary embolism, and muscle wasting. Early mobilization helps reduce these risks by improving circulation and promoting respiratory function [6]. Depending on the surgery type, patients may begin walking or engaging in light activities as soon as they are stable.

- Fluid and electrolyte balance: Proper fluid management is vital for avoiding dehydration, electrolyte imbalances, and renal complications, particularly in patients who have experienced significant blood loss. IV fluids, diuretics, or electrolytes may be adjusted according to the patient's needs [7].

- Nutritional support: The intermediate phase may involve gradual reintroduction of oral feeding or continued nutritional support through IV or enteral routes. Patients recovering from major surgeries often need additional protein and calories to support healing (**Table 1**) [8].

Wound type	Healing method	Care strategy
Primary intention	Sutured/incised wound	Sterile dressing, suture inspection, infection prevention
Secondary intention	Open wound	Regular dressing changes, wound irrigation
Tertiary intention	Delayed closure	Wound debridement, infection control

Table 1.
Types of surgical wounds and their corresponding care strategies.

2.3 Extended postoperative phase

The extended phase of postoperative care takes place after discharge, during which the patient continues recovery at home or in a rehabilitation facility. The goal of this phase is long-term rehabilitation, preventing complications, and ensuring that the patient returns to their normal level of function.

- Follow-up care: Scheduled follow-up visits allow healthcare providers to monitor recovery progress, adjust medications, and address any complications that arise. Depending on the surgery, imaging studies or lab tests may be required to ensure proper healing [9].

- Rehabilitation and physical therapy: Physical therapy is often needed to restore function, strength, and range of motion, especially after orthopedic or neurological surgeries. Tailored rehabilitation programs help prevent long-term disability [10].

- Mental health support: The psychological effects of surgery, such as anxiety, depression, or post-traumatic stress, can delay recovery. Mental health professionals may be involved in the extended postoperative phase to provide counseling and emotional support [11].

3. Pain management in postoperative care

Postoperative pain, if not adequately managed, can lead to complications, including delayed healing, impaired respiratory function, and chronic pain syndromes. Effective pain management improves patient comfort, promotes early mobilization, and facilitates recovery [12].

3.1 Pharmacological pain management

Pharmacological interventions remain the cornerstone of postoperative pain relief. A multimodal approach combining opioids, NSAIDs, local anesthetics, and adjuvant therapies is often employed.

- Opioid analgesics: Opioids, such as morphine, fentanyl, and hydromorphone, are commonly used for moderate to severe pain. While effective, opioids have potential side effects, including respiratory depression, nausea, constipation,

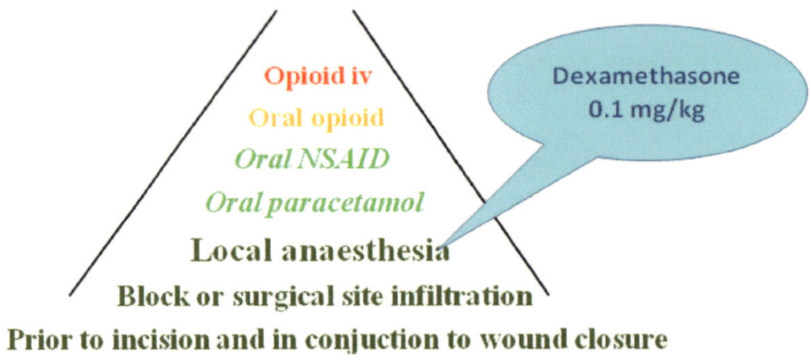

Figure 1.
Commonly used postoperative analgesics.

and risk of dependence. Careful titration and monitoring are essential to balance pain relief with safety (**Figure 1**) [13].

- Nonsteroidal Anti-Inflammatory Drugs (NSAIDs): NSAIDs, such as ibuprofen and ketorolac, are used to manage mild to moderate pain. They work by reducing inflammation, which is often a source of postoperative pain. However, NSAIDs carry a risk of gastrointestinal bleeding and should be used cautiously, particularly in patients with renal impairment [14].

- Local anesthetics: Local anesthetics, such as bupivacaine and lidocaine, can be used for regional nerve blocks or local infiltration to provide targeted pain relief without systemic side effects. Continuous nerve block catheters are increasingly used in major surgeries to provide prolonged pain relief (**Table 2**) [15].

3.1.1 Multimodal analgesia

Multimodal analgesia is an effective strategy for reducing opioid consumption while enhancing pain relief. It combines different types of pain relief methods, such as regional anesthesia, NSAIDs, acetaminophen, and other non-opioid medications. A study in the *Journal of Pain Management* reported that patients receiving multimodal analgesia experienced significantly lower pain scores and required fewer opioids during recovery [16].

- *Local anesthetics*: Administering local anesthetics at the surgical site helps manage pain at the source and reduces the need for systemic medications [17].

Drug type	Example drugs	Indication/Use
Opioids	Morphine, Fentanyl	Moderate to severe pain
NSAIDs	Ibuprofen, Ketorolac	Mild to moderate pain, inflammation
Local anesthetics	Lidocaine, Bupivacaine	Regional blocks, local pain relief

Table 2.
Pharmacological options for postoperative pain management.

- *Cognitive behavioral therapy (CBT)*: CBT, when used alongside pharmacological approaches, can help patients manage pain and reduce postoperative anxiety [18].

3.2 Non-pharmacological pain management

Non-pharmacological methods are often used as adjuncts to pharmacological pain relief. These methods are beneficial because they reduce reliance on medications and help patients cope with pain.

- Cold and heat therapy: Cold therapy (cryotherapy) can reduce swelling and numb pain, particularly in the first 24 to 48 hours after surgery. Heat therapy can be used later to relax muscles and promote circulation [19].

- Cognitive-Behavioral Therapy (CBT): CBT and other psychological interventions can help patients manage pain by changing their perception of it. Techniques such as mindfulness, relaxation training, and guided imagery are often employed [20].

- Physical therapy: Gentle exercises and movement techniques prescribed by physiotherapists can reduce stiffness, improve mobility, and decrease pain associated with immobility [21].

4. Monitoring vital signs and preventing complications

Monitoring vital signs and other physiological parameters is essential in the postoperative period to detect complications early and intervene promptly.

4.1 Cardiovascular monitoring

- Heart rate and blood pressure: Sudden changes in heart rate or blood pressure can signal bleeding, sepsis, or cardiovascular instability. Continuous monitoring is vital in patients recovering from major surgeries, especially those with preexisting cardiovascular conditions [22].

- Central Venous Pressure (CVP): For patients requiring intensive monitoring, especially those with fluid imbalances or heart failure, CVP measurements may be used to assess fluid status and cardiac function.

4.2 Respiratory monitoring

- Oxygen saturation: Postoperative hypoxia can occur due to residual anesthesia effects or respiratory depression from opioid use. Continuous pulse oximetry helps detect hypoxia early, allowing for interventions such as oxygen therapy or respiratory support [23].

- Pulmonary complications: Patients who have undergone thoracic or abdominal surgeries are at an increased risk for pulmonary complications such as atelectasis,

Parameter	Normal range
Oxygen saturation (SpO2)	95–100%
Heart rate	60–100 beats per minute
Blood pressure	90/60 mmHg–120/80 mmHg
Respiratory rate	12–20 breaths per minute

Table 3.
Postoperative monitoring parameters and normal ranges.

pneumonia, and pulmonary embolism. Incentive spirometry, deep breathing exercises, and early mobilization are recommended to reduce these risks (**Table 3**) [24].

5. Wound care and infection prevention

5.1 Wound healing

Effective wound care is essential for preventing infections and promoting healing. Surgical wounds can heal by primary intention (clean incision with sutures) or secondary intention (left open to heal). Proper wound care techniques depend on the wound type and the patient's overall health [25].

- Primary intention: In surgical wounds closed with sutures or staples, keeping the wound clean and dry is critical to prevent infection. Dressings should be changed regularly using sterile techniques.

- Secondary intention: For wounds left to heal on their own, regular cleaning, irrigation, and dressing changes are necessary to promote granulation and tissue growth [26].

5.2 Preventing surgical site infections (SSIs)

Surgical site infections (SSIs) are one of the most common complications in the postoperative period, accounting for up to 20% of healthcare-associated infections [27]. Preventing SSIs requires a combination of intraoperative and postoperative measures.

- Intraoperative measures: Proper sterilization of instruments, antibiotic prophylaxis, and maintaining a sterile field during surgery are critical in reducing the risk of SSIs [28].

- Postoperative measures: Postoperatively, maintaining proper wound care, using sterile dressings, and monitoring for signs of infection (e.g., redness, swelling, and warmth) are essential for preventing SSIs. Early diagnosis and treatment with antibiotics or wound drainage may be required for established infections [29].

6. Rehabilitation and long-term recovery

Rehabilitation is an integral part of postoperative care, especially after major surgeries. Early intervention and a structured rehabilitation plan are essential for restoring function and improving quality of life.

6.1 Physical therapy and functional recovery

Physical therapy is often initiated as early as the immediate postoperative phase. In collaboration with physiotherapists, patients work on strengthening exercises, range-of-motion exercises, and gait training. The goals are to restore function, prevent muscle atrophy, and improve the patient's overall mobility (**Table 4**) [30].

6.2 Psychological support

The psychological impact of surgery and the recovery process should not be overlooked. Patients may experience anxiety, depression, or fear regarding their recovery. Providing emotional support, counseling services, and mental health resources can significantly improve postoperative outcomes [31].

6.3 Nutritional support in postoperative recovery

Nutritional support is often overlooked but plays a crucial role in the healing process after surgery. Postoperative patients have increased metabolic demands, and early nutritional support, through either enteral or parenteral nutrition, can significantly enhance recovery [32]. Malnutrition can lead to delayed wound healing, increased infection risks, and prolonged hospital stays [33].

6.3.1 Types of postoperative nutrition

- Enteral nutrition: Preferred when the gastrointestinal tract is functional, enteral feeding can begin within 24–48 h after surgery. Studies show that early enteral nutrition reduces the risk of infections and shortens hospital stays [34].

- Parenteral nutrition: If enteral nutrition is not possible due to conditions like bowel obstruction or severe gastrointestinal dysfunction, parenteral nutrition is administered intravenously to ensure the patient receives essential nutrients (**Figure 2**) [35].

Surgical procedure	Rehabilitation focus
Joint replacement	Range of motion, strengthening exercises
Spinal surgery	Core stabilization, flexibility training
Abdominal surgery	Breathing exercises, light walking
Cardiac surgery	Cardiovascular conditioning, mobility

Table 4.
Types of postoperative rehabilitation exercises by surgical type.

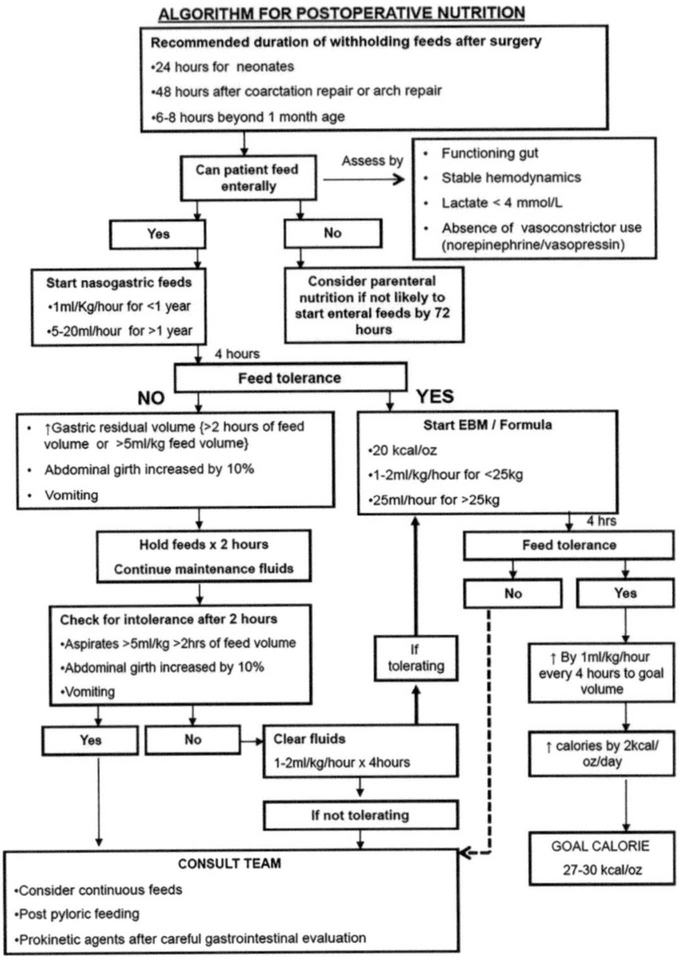

Figure 2.
Nutritional pathways for postoperative patients.

6.4 Pain management techniques

While pharmacological methods, such as opioids and NSAIDs, are commonly used in postoperative pain management, there has been a shift toward multimodal pain management strategies. These strategies reduce opioid reliance and improve patient outcomes [16].

6.4.1 Multimodal analgesia

Multimodal analgesia combines different types of pain relief methods to minimize the use of opioids. These can include regional anesthesia, NSAIDs, acetaminophen, and other non-opioid medications. A study published in the Journal of Pain Management reported that patients receiving multimodal analgesia experienced significantly lower pain scores and required fewer opioids during their recovery [36].

Pain management method	Advantages	Disadvantages
Opioids	Effective for severe pain	Risk of addiction, side effects
NSAIDs	Reduces inflammation	Risk of gastrointestinal issues
Local anesthetics	Targets pain at the source	Short duration
Cognitive behavioral therapy	Reduces anxiety and pain	Requires time and patient effort

Table 5.
Comparison of pain management methods in postoperative care.

- Local anesthetics: Administering local anesthetics at the surgical site helps manage pain at the source and reduces the need for systemic medications [17].

- Cognitive Behavioral Therapy (CBT): Used alongside pharmacological approaches, CBT has been shown to help patients better manage their pain and reduce anxiety postoperatively (**Table 5**) [18].

7. Common postoperative complications

Postoperative complications are relatively common, and their early detection and management are key to improving patient outcomes. Complications range from mild, such as nausea and vomiting, to life-threatening conditions like deep vein thrombosis (DVT) or pulmonary embolism (PE).

7.1 Cardiovascular complications

Cardiovascular complications, including myocardial infarction (MI), stroke, and deep vein thrombosis (DVT), pose significant risks after surgery, particularly in high-risk patients [37].

- DVT and pulmonary embolism: Postoperative immobility increases the risk of DVT and PE. Early mobilization, use of compression stockings, and prophylactic anticoagulation therapy are critical measures to prevent these complications [38].

- Postoperative myocardial infarction (POMI): Cardiovascular monitoring is essential in high-risk patients to prevent POMI. According to the American Heart Journal, 3–5% of postoperative patients develop some form of cardiovascular complication, particularly after major surgeries [39].

7.2 Respiratory complications

Respiratory complications, such as pneumonia, atelectasis, and respiratory failure, are common after surgeries involving general anesthesia. These complications are more prevalent in elderly patients and those with pre-existing pulmonary conditions [40].

- Atelectasis: The collapse of alveoli can lead to inadequate oxygenation postoperatively. Techniques like incentive spirometry and chest physiotherapy are often employed to prevent or resolve atelectasis [41].
- Postoperative pneumonia: Preventive measures include early ambulation, breathing exercises, and prophylactic antibiotics in high-risk patients [42].

8. Enhanced recovery after surgery (ERAS) protocols

Enhanced Recovery After Surgery (ERAS) protocols are a comprehensive, multidisciplinary approach to perioperative care that aims to improve surgical outcomes, reduce complications, and promote faster recovery. Developed in the late 1990s, these protocols are based on evidence-based strategies that optimize patient care across the preoperative, intraoperative, and postoperative stages. By implementing these guidelines, healthcare providers can enhance recovery times, reduce hospital stays, and improve overall patient satisfaction [43].

8.1 Key principles of ERAS protocols

ERAS protocols emphasize reducing the physical and psychological stress of surgery through an integrated approach. The following principles are fundamental to ERAS:

Preoperative optimization:

- Patient education: Informing patients about the surgical process, potential risks, and the recovery plan. This includes setting realistic expectations and encouraging patient involvement in their own care [44].
- Nutritional optimization: Ensuring patients are nutritionally prepared for surgery. Malnutrition can lead to delayed healing and increased risk of complications. Carbohydrate loading (instead of fasting) just before surgery has been shown to improve outcomes [45].
- Minimizing fasting: ERAS protocols advocate for shortened fasting periods (often only 6 h for solids and 2 h for liquids) before surgery, which helps maintain energy stores and reduces insulin resistance [46].
- Smoking and alcohol cessation: Patients are encouraged to stop smoking and limit alcohol intake before surgery, as both can impair wound healing and increase complication risks (**Table 6**) [47].

Metric	Traditional Care	ERAS Protocols
Time to mobilization	24–48 hours after surgery	4–6 hours after surgery
Time to oral nutrition	24–48 hours after surgery	Within 24 hours
Hospital stay	5–10 days	3–5 days
Postoperative complication rate	Higher	Reduced

Table 6.
Comparison of traditional postoperative care vs. ERAS protocols.

Intraoperative care:

- Minimally invasive surgical techniques: Whenever possible, less invasive procedures are preferred as they cause less tissue damage and reduce postoperative pain, which contributes to faster recovery [48].

- Multimodal analgesia: This strategy minimizes opioid use by combining various analgesics and pain management techniques (such as NSAIDs, regional anesthesia, and local anesthetics). By reducing opioid dependency, patients are less likely to experience opioid-related side effects like constipation, nausea, and respiratory depression [49].

- Fluid management: Optimal fluid balance is critical in ERAS protocols. Avoiding both dehydration and overhydration is key, as excess fluid can increase the risk of postoperative complications such as edema and impaired wound healing [50].

- Temperature regulation: Maintaining normal body temperature during surgery can prevent complications such as wound infections and cardiovascular stress [51].

Postoperative care:

- Early mobilization: ERAS emphasizes early movement (within hours after surgery) to prevent complications like deep vein thrombosis (DVT), pulmonary embolism (PE), and muscle atrophy. Early ambulation improves circulation, lung function, and gastrointestinal motility [52].

- Early enteral nutrition: Initiating oral intake as early as possible (within 24 hours postoperatively) helps to restore gut function, reduce the risk of infections, and promote healing. Studies have shown that early enteral feeding shortens hospital stays and lowers the incidence of complications such as wound infections and pneumonia [53].

- Pain control: As previously discussed, a multimodal approach to pain management is used to provide effective analgesia with minimal reliance on opioids. This enhances recovery by minimizing opioid-related side effects and allowing patients to be more active and cooperative with their rehabilitation programs [54].

- Prevention of postoperative complications: Proactive measures are employed to prevent common complications such as DVT, PE, atelectasis, and infections. For example, mechanical prophylaxis with compression stockings or pharmacological prophylaxis (e.g., anticoagulants) are used to prevent thromboembolic events [55].

- Psychological support: Anxiety and stress can negatively impact recovery. ERAS encourages psychological support, including cognitive behavioral therapy (CBT), mindfulness techniques, and open communication between patients and healthcare providers [56].

8.2 Benefits of ERAS protocols

ERAS has been associated with numerous benefits across various types of surgeries, including colorectal, orthopedic, cardiac, and gynecological procedures. The primary advantages include:

- Reduced postoperative complications: ERAS protocols have consistently been shown to reduce the incidence of complications such as infections, thromboembolic events, and cardiovascular issues. This is due to the emphasis on early mobilization, proper pain control, and fluid management [57].
- Shortened hospital stay: Studies have demonstrated that ERAS protocols can reduce hospital stay durations by 2 to 3 days on average. By promoting early mobilization, nutrition, and pain management, patients recover more quickly and are discharged sooner [58].
- Improved patient outcomes: By reducing the physical and psychological stress associated with surgery, ERAS improves overall patient outcomes. Patients experience less pain, recover mobility faster, and regain normal gastrointestinal function sooner [59].
- Cost-effectiveness: Shortened hospital stays and fewer complications lead to lower healthcare costs, making ERAS protocols financially beneficial for both healthcare providers and patients [60].

8.3 Evidence supporting ERAS protocols

Numerous studies support the effectiveness of ERAS protocols. For instance, a study published in The British Journal of Surgery reported that ERAS reduced postoperative complications by up to 50% and shortened hospital stays by 2–3 days [59, 60]. Similarly, a meta-analysis of over 5000 patients found that ERAS protocols significantly reduced morbidity rates without increasing readmissions [61].

A systematic review of colorectal surgeries, which are a primary area of ERAS implementation, found that patients on ERAS pathways experienced fewer postoperative ileus episodes, reduced narcotic use, and faster return of bowel function compared to traditional care approaches [62].

8.4 ERAS in special populations

ERAS protocols can be adapted for various surgical populations, including high-risk patients such as the elderly, those with chronic illnesses, and patients undergoing complex surgeries. Key considerations include:

- Elderly patients: Elderly patients are at increased risk of postoperative complications due to comorbidities and decreased physiological reserves. ERAS protocols tailored for this population focus on optimizing preoperative health, minimizing invasive procedures, and closely monitoring fluid and pain management to avoid delirium and other age-related complications [63].

- Cancer patients: In oncological surgeries, ERAS can help reduce immunosuppression and accelerate recovery, allowing patients to resume adjuvant treatments like chemotherapy sooner [64].

- Cardiac surgery patients: ERAS protocols for cardiac surgeries emphasize early extubation, multimodal analgesia, and early mobilization to reduce the risk of pulmonary complications and cardiac events [65].

8.5 Barriers to ERAS implementation

While the benefits of ERAS are well-documented, several barriers can impede its widespread adoption:

- Lack of awareness or training: Some healthcare providers may not be fully aware of ERAS protocols or lack the training necessary to implement them effectively [66].

- Resistance to change: Traditional surgical practices are deeply ingrained in some institutions, leading to resistance to the adoption of new methodologies [67].

- Resource constraints: Implementing ERAS protocols may require additional resources, such as specialized equipment for minimally invasive surgery or training for staff. In some healthcare settings, these resources may be limited [68].

8.6 Future directions

ERAS protocols continue to evolve as new evidence emerges and surgical techniques advance. Key areas of future development include:

- Personalized ERAS pathways: As more data is collected on ERAS outcomes, the protocols may become increasingly personalized to account for individual patient characteristics, such as age, comorbidities, and specific surgical risks [69].

- Integration of technology: Advances in digital health, such as remote monitoring, artificial intelligence (AI), and telemedicine, could further enhance ERAS protocols by enabling real-time data collection, personalized interventions, and more effective postoperative monitoring [70].

9. Innovations in postoperative care

Technological advancements are revolutionizing postoperative care. These innovations aim to improve patient monitoring, provide real-time data for clinicians, and enhance recovery outcomes [71].

9.1 Remote monitoring technologies

Wearable devices and remote monitoring systems allow continuous monitoring of vital signs (e.g., heart rate, oxygen saturation) outside the hospital setting. This can lead to earlier detection of complications and reduced readmissions [72].

Telemedicine platforms also provide remote consultations, enabling healthcare providers to adjust treatment plans without requiring the patient to return to the hospital.

9.2 Artificial intelligence in postoperative care

Artificial intelligence (AI) has the potential to predict postoperative complications and personalize care based on the patient's unique data [48]. Machine learning algorithms can analyze data from past surgical patients to predict the likelihood of complications like infections or respiratory issues. AI-driven systems are also being used to optimize pain management strategies [73].

10. Conclusion

The evolving field of postoperative care is grounded in comprehensive strategies that encompass immediate recovery, long-term rehabilitation, and patient-centered interventions. Advances in technology, pain management, infection prevention, and rehabilitation programs have significantly reduced postoperative morbidity and mortality. Going forward, innovations like ERAS protocols, AI-driven care, and telemedicine will continue to shape the future of postoperative recovery. Ensuring that healthcare providers are equipped with updated knowledge and tools is critical for the continued improvement of patient outcomes.

Acknowledgements

In the creation of this manuscript, AI-based tools were utilized to aid in refining the structure and improving the flow of the text. As the author is a non-native English speaker, these tools were employed to ensure that the language was accessible and coherent for an international audience. However, the scientific content, research, and conclusions presented are entirely the author's own. The AI tools were used solely as linguistic aids to enhance clarity and style, with no influence on the generation of ideas or academic content. Their role was limited to ensuring that the manuscript met the stylistic expectations of a broad readership.

Author details

Visar Disha
Faculty of Medicine, University of Prishtina, Prishtina, Kosovo

*Address all correspondence to: dishavisar@gmail.com

IntechOpen

© 2025 The Author(s). Licensee IntechOpen. This chapter is distributed under the terms of the Creative Commons Attribution License (http://creativecommons.org/licenses/by/4.0), which permits unrestricted use, distribution, and reproduction in any medium, provided the original work is properly cited. (cc) BY

References

[1] O'Neill F, Carter E, Pink N, Smith I. Routine preoperative tests for elective surgery: Summary of updated NICE guidance. BMJ. 2016;**354**:i3292

[2] Patel S et al. Anesthesia recovery and airway management. Anesthesiology Review. 2022;**39**(4):121-130

[3] Shaydakov ME, Tuma F. Operative Risk. In: StatPearls [Internet]. Treasure Island (FL): StatPearls Publishing; 2024. 2023

[4] Eller OC, Willits AB, Young EE, Baumbauer KM. Pharmacological and non-pharmacological therapeutic interventions for the treatment of spinal cord injury-induced pain. Frontiers in Pain Research (Lausanne). 2022;**3**:991736. DOI: 10.3389/fpain.2022.991736

[5] Mills GH, Groves J. Postoperative care. In: Fundamentals of Anaesthesia. 5th ed. Oxford: Oxford University Press; 2016. DOI: 10.1093/med/9780199665549.003.0083

[6] Euliano TY, Gravenstein JS, Gravenstein N, Gravenstein D. Post-operative care. In: Clinical Management. Cambridge University Press; 2011. DOI: 10.1017/CBO9780511975771.013

[7] Tyson E, Creagh-Brown B. Postoperative care. Medicine. 2018;**46**(12):750-753. DOI: 10.1016/j.mpmed.2018.09.003

[8] Falk SA. Postoperative care. Anesthesiology Clinics. 2012;**30**(3):xi-xii. DOI: 10.1016/j.anclin.2012.07.013

[9] SARVIS, CONNIE. Postoperative wound care. Nursing. 2006;**36**(12):56-57. DOI: 10.1097/00152193-200612000-00044

[10] Kelly DF. Neurosurgical Postoperative Care. Neurosurgery Clinics of North America. 1994;**5**(4):789-810. DOI: 10.1016/s1042-3680(18)30501-1

[11] Adatia I, Beghetti M. Immediate postoperative care. Cardiology in the Young. 2009;**19**(S1):23-27. DOI: 10.1017/s1047951109003916

[12] Rees NW. Nursing Management of Postoperative Pain: Perceived Care and Actual Practice (Thesis). Curtin University; 2000 Available from: http://hdl.handle.net/20.500.11937/1235

[13] Pucher P. Structural and Care Process Improvement of Ward-Based Postoperative Care to Optimise Surgical Outcomes (Thesis). London: Imperial College; 2014. Available from: http://hdl.handle.net/10044/1/24994

[14] Delaney CP. Postoperative ileus. Oxford: Oxford University Press; 2010

[15] Halpern NA, McElhinney AJ, Greenstein R. Postoperative sepsis. Critical Care Medicine. 1990;**18**(Supplement):S200. DOI: 10.1097/00003246-199012001-00049

[16] Ling ML, Apisarnthanarak A, Abbas A, et al. APSIC guidelines for the prevention of surgical site infections. Antimicrobial Resistance and Infection Control. 2019;**8**:174

[17] National Collaborating Centre for Women's and Children's Health Guideline Development Group. Surgical Site Infection: Prevention and Treatment of Surgical Site Infection. London (UK): National Collaborating Centre for Women's and Children's Health; 2008, (updated 2019). Available from: https://

www.nice.org.uk/guidance/ng125/evidence/october-2008-full-guideline-pdf-6727105694 [Accessed: June 08, 2020]

[18] Brett K, Severn M. Nasal Decolonization for the Prevention of Surgical Site Infections: A Review of Clinical Effectiveness and Cost-Effectiveness [CADTH Rapid Response Report: Summary with Critical Appraisal]. Ottawa (ON): CADTH; 2020

[19] Hegtvedt AK. Intraoperative and postoperative patient care. Oral and Maxillofacial Surgery Clinics of North America. 1990;**2**(4):857-868. DOI: 10.1016/s1042-3699(20)30468-4

[20] Pilipczuk O, Eidenzon D, Kosenko O. Patient Postoperative Care Data Visualization. International Journal of Computer Applications. 15, 2016;**156**(7):27-33. DOI: 10.5120/ijca2016912469

[21] Lee DK, Kim YH, Kim JH. Postoperative care of geriatric patients. Journal of the Korean Medical Association. 2017;**60**(5):384. DOI: 10.5124/jkma.2017.60.5.384

[22] McQuay H, Moore A. The concept of postoperative care. Current Opinion in Anaesthesiology. 1997;**10**(5):369-373. DOI: 10.1097/00001503-199710000-00018

[23] Sarwer DB. The importance of postoperative care. Bariatric Nursing and Surgical Patient Care. 2008;**3**(2):89-91. DOI: 10.1089/bar.2008.9983

[24] Myers EC. Evaluation of a Patient-Controlled Approach to Postoperative Pain Relief (Thesis). Glasgow Caledonian University; 1993. Available from: http://ethos.bl.uk/OrderDetails.do?uin=uk.bl.ethos.335359

[25] International Surgical Outcomes Study Group. Global patient outcomes after elective surgery: Prospective cohort study in 27 low-, middle- and high-income countries. British Journal of Anaesthesia. 2016;**117**(5):601-609

[26] Devitt P. Postoperative management. In: Smith JA, Kaye AH, Christophi C, Brown WA, editors. 1st ed. 2019

[27] Suzuki S. Oxygen administration for postoperative surgical patients: A narrative review. Journal of Intensive Care. 2020;**8**:79

[28] Berrios-Torres SI, Umscheid CA, Bratzler DW, et al. Centers for Disease Control and Prevention guideline for the prevention of surgical site infection, 2017. JAMA Surgery. 2017;**152**(8):784-791

[29] Canadian Patient Safety Institute. Canadian Surgical Site Infection Prevention Audit Month [Recap Report]. Ottawa (ON): Canadian Patient Safety Institute; 2016. Available from: https://www.patientsafetyinstitute.ca/en/toolsResources/Documents/SSI%20Audit%202016_Recap%20Report%20EN.pdf [Accessed: May 22, 2020]

[30] Anderson D, Sexton D. Overview of control measures for prevention of surgical site infection in adults. In: Post TW, editor. UpToDate. Waltham (MA): UpToDate; 2020. Available from: www.uptodate.com [Accessed: June 15, 2020]

[31] Umscheid CA, Mitchell MD, Doshi JA, Agarwal R, Williams K, Brennan PJ. Estimating the proportion of healthcare-associated infections that are reasonably preventable and the related mortality and costs. Infection Control and Hospital Epidemiology. 2011;**32**(2):101-114

[32] Li Y, Severn M. Nasal Decolonization for the Prevention of Surgical Site Infections: Clinical Effectiveness, Cost-Effectiveness, and Guidelines. [CADTH Rapid Response Report: Reference List]. CADTH: Ottawa (ON); 2020. Available from: https://cadth.ca/nasal-decolonization-prevention-surgical-site-infectionsclinical-effectiveness-cost-effectiveness [Accessed: April 28, 2020]

[33] Liberati A, Altman DG, Tetzlaff J, et al. The PRISMA statement for reporting systematic reviews and meta-analyses of studies that evaluate health care interventions: Explanation and elaboration. Journal of Clinical Epidemiology. 2009;**62**(10):e1-e34

[34] Allegranzi B, Bischoff P, Kubilay Z, et al. Global Guidelines for the Prevention of Surgical Site Infection. Geneva, Switzerland: World Health Organization (WHO); 2016. Available from: https://apps.who.int/iris/bitstream/handle/10665/250680/9789241549882-eng.pdf?sequence=8 [Accessed: April 28, 2020]

[35] NICE. Surgical Site Infections: Prevention and Treatment [Clinical Guideline NG125]. London (UK): National Institute for Health and Care Excellence; 2019. Available from: https://www.nice.org.uk/guidance/ng125/resources/surgical-site-infections-prevention-and-treatment-pdf-66141660564421 [Accessed: April 28, 2020]

[36] Ban KA, Minei JP, Laronga C, et al. American College of Surgeons and surgical infection society: Surgical site infection guidelines, 2016 update. Journal of the American College of Surgeons. 2017;**224**(1):59-74

[37] Edmiston CE Jr, Lee CJ, Krepel CJ, et al. Evidence for a standardized preadmission showering regimen to achieve maximal antiseptic skin surface concentrations of chlorhexidine gluconate, 4%, in surgical patients. JAMA Surgery. 2015;**150**(11):1027-1033

[38] Nelson RL, Gladman E, Barbateskovic M. Antimicrobial prophylaxis for colorectal surgery. Cochrane Database of Systematic Reviews. 2014;**5**:Cd001181

[39] Lefebvre A, Saliou P, Lucet JC, et al. Preoperative hair removal and surgical site infections: Network meta-analysis of randomized controlled trials. The Journal of Hospital Infection. 2015;**91**(2):100-108

[40] Tanner J, Norrie P, Melen K. Preoperative hair removal to reduce surgical site infection. Cochrane Database of Systematic Reviews. 2011;**11**:Cd004122

[41] Allegranzi B, Bischoff P, de Jonge S, et al. New WHO recommendations on preoperative measures for surgical site infection prevention: An evidence-based global perspective. The Lancet Infectious Diseases. 2016;**16**(12):e276-e287

[42] van Rijen M, Bonten M, Wenzel R, Kluytmans J. Mupirocin ointment for preventing Staphylococcus aureus infections in nasal carriers. Cochrane Database of Systematic Reviews. 2008;**4**:Cd006216

[43] Pofahl WE, Goettler CE, Ramsey KM, Cochran MK, Nobles DL, Rotondo MF. Active surveillance screening of MRSA and eradication of the carrier state decreases surgical-site infections caused by MRSA. Journal of the American College of Surgeons. 2009;**208**(5):981-986

[44] Maiwald M, Chan ES. The forgotten role of alcohol: A systematic review and

meta-analysis of the clinical efficacy and perceived role of chlorhexidine in skin antisepsis. PLoS One. 2012;7(9):e44277

[45] Dumville JC, McFarlane E, Edwards P, Lipp A, Holmes A. Preoperative skin antiseptics for preventing surgical wound infections after clean surgery. Cochrane Database of Systematic Reviews. 2013;**3**:Cd003949

[46] Anderson DJ, Podgorny K, Berríos-Torres SI, et al. Strategies to prevent surgical site infections in acute care hospitals: 2014 update. Infection Control and Hospital Epidemiology. 2014;**35**(6):605-627

[47] Webster J, Osborne S. Preoperative bathing or showering with skin antiseptics to prevent surgical site infection. Cochrane Database of Systematic Reviews. 2012;**9**

[48] Walsh EE, Greene L, Kirshner R. Sustained reduction in methicillin-resistant Staphylococcus aureus wound infections after cardiothoracic surgery. Archives of Internal Medicine. 2011;**171**(1):68-73

[49] Schweizer ML, Chiang H-Y, Septimus E, et al. Association of a bundled intervention with surgical site infections among patients undergoing cardiac, hip, or knee surgery. Journal of the American Medical Association. 2015;**313**(21):2162-2171

[50] Awad SS, Palacio CH, Subramanian A, et al. Implementation of a methicillin-resistant Staphylococcus aureus (MRSA) prevention bundle results in decreased MRSA surgical site infections. American Journal of Surgery. 2009;**198**(5):607-610

[51] Reichman DE, Greenberg JA. Reducing surgical site infections: A review. Reviews in Obstetrics and Gynecology. 2009;**2**(4):212-221

[52] Mangram AJ, Horan TC, Pearson ML, Silver LC, Jarvis WR. Guideline for prevention of surgical site infection, 1999. Centers for Disease Control and Prevention (CDC) hospital infection control practices advisory committee. American Journal of Infection Control. 1999;**27**(2):97-132

[53] Sidhwa F, Itani KMF. Skin preparation before surgery: Options and evidence. Surgical Infections. 2015;**16**(1):14-23

[54] Cataife G, Weinberg DA, Wong HH, Kahn KL. The effect of surgical care improvement project (SCIP) compliance on surgical site infections (SSI). Medical Care. 2014;**52**(2 Suppl. 1):S66-S73

[55] Bratzler DW, Dellinger EP, Olsen KM, et al. Clinical practice guidelines for antimicrobial prophylaxis in surgery. Surgical Infections. 2013;**14**(1):73-156

[56] Vriesendorp TM, Morélis QJ, DeVries JH, Legemate DA, Hoekstra JBL. Early post-operative glucose levels are an independent risk factor for infection after peripheral vascular surgery. A retrospective study. European Journal of Vascular and Endovascular Surgery. 2004;**28**(5):520-525

[57] Lazar HL, McDonnell MM, Chipkin S, Fitzgerald C, Bliss C, Cabral H. Effects of aggressive versus moderate glycemic control on clinical outcomes in diabetic coronary artery bypass graft patients. Annals of Surgery. 2011;**254**(3):458-464

[58] Kwon S, Thompson R, Dellinger P, Yanez D, Farrohki E, Flum D. Importance of perioperative glycemic

control in general surgery: A report from the surgical care and outcomes assessment program. Annals of Surgery. 2013;**257**(1):8-14

[59] Kotagal M, Symons RG, Hirsch IB, et al. Perioperative hyperglycemia and risk of adverse events among patients with and without diabetes. Annals of Surgery. 2015;**261**(1):97-103

[60] Kirdemir P, Yildirim V, Kiris I, et al. Does continuous insulin therapy reduce postoperative supraventricular tachycardia incidence after coronary artery bypass operations in diabetic patients? Journal of Cardiothoracic and Vascular Anesthesia. 2008;**22**(3):383-387

[61] Grey NJ, Perdrizet GA. Reduction of nosocomial infections in the surgical intensive-care unit by strict glycemic control. Endocrine Practice. 2004;**10**(Suppl. 2):46-52

[62] Emam IA, Allan A, Eskander K, et al. Our experience of controlling diabetes in the peri-operative period of patients who underwent cardiac surgery. Diabetes Research and Clinical Practice. 2010;**88**(3):242-246

[63] Desai SP, Henry LL, Holmes SD, et al. Strict versus liberal target range for perioperative glucose in patients undergoing coronary artery bypass grafting: A prospective randomized controlled trial. The Journal of Thoracic and Cardiovascular Surgery. 2012;**143**(2):318-325

[64] Chan RPC, Galas FRBG, Hajjar LA, Bello CN, Piccioni MA, Auler Jr JOC. Intensive perioperative glucose control does not improve outcomes of patients submitted to open-heart surgery: A randomized controlled trial. Clinics. 2009;**64**(1):51-60

[65] Bratzler DW, Hunt DR. The surgical infection prevention and surgical care improvement projects: National initiatives to improve outcomes for patients having surgery. Clinical Infectious Diseases. 2006;**43**(3):322-330

[66] Bilotta F, Spinelli A, Giovannini F, Doronzio A, Delfini R, Rosa G. The effect of intensive insulin therapy on infection rate, vasospasm, neurologic outcome, and mortality in neurointensive care unit after intracranial aneurysm clipping in patients with acute subarachnoid hemorrhage: A randomized prospective pilot trial. Journal of Neurosurgical Anesthesiology. 2007;**19**(3):156-160

[67] Ata A, Lee J, Bestle SL, Desemone J, Stain SC. Postoperative hyperglycemia and surgical site infection in general surgery patients. Archives of Surgery. 2010;**145**(9):858-864

[68] Berrios-Torres SI, Umscheid CA, Bratzler DW, et al. Healthcare infection control practices advisory committee. Centers for Disease Control and Prevention guideline for the prevention of surgical site infection, 2017 (supplementary online content). JAMA Surgery. 2017;**152**(8)

[69] Renner J, Moikow L, Lorenzen U. Enhanced recovery after surgery (ERAS): Less is more : What must be considered from an anesthesiological perspective? Der Chirurg. 2021;**92**(5):421-427

[70] de Boer HD, Fawcett WJ, Scott MJ. Enhanced recovery after surgery: The road to improve peri-operative care globally. European Journal of Anaesthesiology. 2021;**38**(9):905-907

[71] Moningi S, Patki A, Padhy N, Ramachandran G. Enhanced recovery after surgery: An anesthesiologist's perspective.

Journal of Anaesthesiology Clinical Pharmacology. 2019;**35**(Suppl.1):S5-S13

[72] Byrnes A, Banks M, Mudge A, et al. Enhanced recovery after surgery as an auditing framework or identifying improvements to perioperative nutrition care of older surgical patients. European Journal of Clinical Nutrition. 2018;**72**:913-916

[73] Ljungqvist O, Scott M, Fearon KC. Enhanced recovery after surgery: A review. JAMA Surgery. 2017;**152**:292-298